THE
NEW SCIENCE
OF
OVERCOMING ARTHRITIS

THE
NEW SCIENCE
OF
OVERCOMING
ARTHRITIS

Prevent or Reverse Your Pain,
Discomfort, and Limitations

C. THOMAS VANGSNESS, JR., MD
with Greg Ptacek

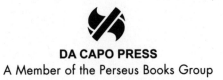

DA CAPO PRESS
A Member of the Perseus Books Group

Designed by Cynthia Young

Cataloging-in-Publication data for this book is
available from the Library of Congress.

First Da Capo Press edition 2013
ISBN: 978-0-7382-1722-2 (paperback)
ISBN: 978-0-7382-1723-9 (e-book)

Published by Da Capo Press
A Member of the Perseus Books Group
www.dacapopress.com

Note: The information in this book is true and complete to the best of our knowledge. This book is intended only as an informative guide for those wishing to know more about health issues. In no way is this book intended to replace, countermand, or conflict with the advice given to you by your own physician. The ultimate decision concerning care should be made between you and your doctor. We strongly recommend you follow his or her advice. Information in this book is general and is offered with no guarantees on the part of the authors or Da Capo Press. The authors and publisher disclaim all liability in connection with the use of this book. The names and identifying details of people associated with events described in this book have been changed. Any similarity to actual persons is coincidental.

Da Capo Press books are available at special discounts for bulk purchases in the U.S. by corporations, institutions, and other organizations. For more information, please contact the Special Markets Department at the Perseus Books Group, 2300 Chestnut Street, Suite 200, Philadelphia, PA, 19103 or call (800) 810-4145, ext. 5000, or e-mail special.markets@ perseusbooks.com.

10 9 8 7 6 5 4 3 2

To my family and my four children
for inspiring me every day,
to my students, residents, and fellows
for sharing with me the joy of learning, and
to my patients who strive to achieve
their optimal quality of life
through an active, healthy lifestyle.

Contents

Introduction

Arthritis—we hear about it every day. Take this medicine or that supplement, and you will feel better and live free of pain once again. Marketed with buckets full of cash from international pharmaceutical corporations, arthritis pills are a $40-billion-a-year business, which is why TV is saturated with commercials for arthritis pain relief.

But what do we really know about this disease? Just what is arthritis?

Here's one sure bet about you and arthritis: you're very likely to suffer from some form of it. In fact, if you live to age seventy-five, you have a 75 percent chance of suffering from osteoarthritis, the most prevalent form of the disease.

As I'll discuss in the coming pages, arthritis is actually many different afflictions, some only remotely related. But they all share a common symptom: inflammation around the joint, causing pain, swelling, and stiffness.

In this book, I'll share with you my thirty years of experience as an orthopedic surgeon and clinician and my more recent cutting-edge stem cell research that offers the hope of cellular regeneration of cartilage—the holy grail of arthritis treatment. Imagine if one day soon your doctor wouldn't prescribe a pill to relieve your aching knee but instead injected a serum that would not only eliminate the pain and inflammation but also possibly reverse the effects of arthritis!

The Arthritis Epidemic

First, however, let's put arthritis into perspective. For the patient, arthritis means suffering the symptoms—aches and pains around joints—on a daily basis. Even worse, for the majority of sufferers, arthritis limits their common everyday activities and decreases the quality of their lives.

In fact, arthritis is the most common chronic disease in our society. It's more common than heart disease, cancer, asthma, hypertension, or diabetes. It ranks as the leading cause of disability among people age sixty-five and older, but it is also a major cause of work-related disability.

Currently, approximately fifty million adults in the United States (about one in six) are affected by arthritis, but this number is predicted to increase to sixty to seventy million by the year 2030.

This is a problem of epidemic proportions, and if nothing else changed, this alone clearly makes arthritis one of the most serious health problems in our society. But there are two disturbing new trends that underscore that the problem is getting worse, not better: the overall rate of osteoarthritis is increasing, and the age of sufferers is decreasing.

Decreasing Age, Increasing Number of Sufferers

While most chronic diseases in America are on a slow decline, arthritis is on a steady increase. Despite its reputation as a disease of old age, the average age of osteoarthritis onset has fallen to forty-seven, and about three out of every five people with arthritis are under sixty-five years of age.

In other words, a greater proportion of people in the United States are suffering from arthritis, and they are suffering at a younger age, than a decade ago. I am seeing this in my own practice—a huge surge of patients exhibiting common symptoms of arthritis at younger ages than was the case twenty or even ten years ago.

Societal Costs

The growing number of arthritis sufferers comes at a tremendous price for society. Arthritis-related expenditures for just one person—lost wages, medical treatment, and other related expenses—can come to more than $150,000 in his or her lifetime. Total costs from arthritis in 2012 are estimated to be approximately $81 billion, with that figure expected to rise dramatically in the next two decades as the baby boom generation comes into its senior years. Adults age sixty-five and older are approximately 13 percent of the US population, yet they accounted for over one-third of the total dollars spent on personal health care.

Although nearly a hundred forms of arthritis affect our population, osteoarthritis is by far the most prominent, responsible for nearly half of all cases. More than 90 percent of osteoarthritis patients report functional limitations in their daily activities. The loss of mobility can make it difficult or impossible to carry out ordinary life activities such as exercising, grocery shopping, house cleaning, gardening, and even dressing oneself. This loss of function can lead to lost wages, job transfers, and even unemployment.

Osteoarthritis accounts for approximately forty million physicians' visits and half a million hospitalizations a year. Patients with symptomatic osteoarthritis use twice as much medical care as patients without arthritis. Other expenses associated with arthritis, including behavioral (lifestyle) changes and adaptations such as change of residence, transportation difficulties, over-the-counter medication, medicines not regulated by the US Food and Drug Administration (FDA), and assistive devices for personal care, only add to the burden. We can anticipate that osteoarthritis-related costs alone will approach $282 billion annually by 2030.

Silent Epidemic

We can take steps to reduce our chances of being affected by arthritis. It is my hope that the facts, figures, analysis, and recommendations presented in this book will reveal to you the problem—which is truly of epidemic proportions—that we face in combating the disease. More important, I'll provide you with concrete ways to fight the disease, based on the very latest in scientific information.

We'll look at the many different types of arthritis and their causes. We will narrow down exactly what people suffering from arthritis can do to help themselves. This will include discussions of both traditional and alternative approaches to the disease, including exercise, weight loss, joint conditioning, currently available drugs, and alternative therapies. Finally, we'll take a look at seemingly futuristic treatments involving stem cells, genes, bionics, and biogenic drugs, all of which are already being used on patients.

While, as we've seen, arthritis imposes tremendous costs on the individual and society, affecting almost all of us either directly or indirectly, osteoarthritis gets scant attention from the news media and a fraction of government funding for research compared to other chronic diseases. It's as if no one is listening. This book aims to turn up the volume on the problem, look beyond the TV commercials peddling pain relief, and make it impossible to ignore this silent epidemic any longer.

1

ARTHRITIS 101

Arthritis is the nation's leading cause of disability, affecting one in six adults in the United States. If you are over fifty-five years of age, you have a 75 percent chance of developing arthritis in your lifetime. By the time you're seventy-nine years old, you're virtually guaranteed of having some arthritis symptoms.

These numbers are daunting, but the real tragedy lies with actual arthritis sufferers such as my patient Mrs. Dodd, an older woman who in ten short years progressed from having minor aches and pains in her hips to being almost completely disabled by arthritis. Today, hobbled by the disease, she relies on a walker and a motorized scooter to carry out the smallest of everyday tasks.

Even though arthritis is affecting more and more of us, the condition is widely misunderstood. I'm reminded of the reality-TV show called *The Pitch,* a real-life version of *Mad Men,* in which two agencies compete for an actual advertising account. One episode revolved around the decision by the Juvenile Diabetes Research Foundation to change its name because, contrary to what was originally thought, most of the sufferers are actually adults. Arthritis has a similar identity problem. Just about every aspect of arthritis is clouded by uncertainty, misinformation, and myth, including how to define it, what its causes are, how best to treat it, and how to predict its course. In my experience, patients who become knowledgeable about their symptoms and the specific diagnosis of their arthritis are most successful in alleviating many of the anxieties associated with arthritic symptoms and are able to live to the fullest within the confines of the disease. In an attempt to demystify the disease, in this chapter I'll outline the basic science of arthritis, explain why it is not one disease but many, and describe and illustrate the anatomy of healthy human joints and their arthritic counterparts. Osteoarthritis, which constitutes more than 90 percent of all cases in the United States, will be the focus of this book.

An Ancient Term for Many Diseases

The term *arthritis* derives from the Greek *arthron,* "joint," and *-itis,* "inflammation." Arthritis has come to be known as simple inflammation about any joint, but that is like saying that any illness that involves a fever is called a fever disease.

To the patient, a diagnosis of arthritis means suffering with swelling, stiffness, and aches and pains around the joint, bones, and muscles on a daily basis. Pain and loss of function are the main symptoms that bring sufferers to a doctor's office for treatment. Unfortunately, by the time you feel the pain, it's usually too late. The permanent damage is already done. Imaging procedures and biochemical marker analyses need to be improved so that we can reliably describe the disease process, diagnose the disease at an early stage, classify patients according to their prognosis, and follow the course of the disease and treatment effectiveness.

Arthritis is really a generic term incorporating a number of varied symptoms. There are many causes of arthritis and more than one hundred types of arthritis, with newer subdivisions being discovered every year. Further, the treatments for each type of the disease are different. Modern technology has allowed us to diagnose and treat the various forms of arthritis in a very sophisticated and intelligent fashion. Today, each type of arthritis can be diagnosed and defined for the patient so that treatment and lifestyle plans can be tailored to the individual.

Because of the wide range in types of arthritis, it is best to divide the disease into two simple categories: osteoarthritis and inflammatory arthritis. While many of the symptoms are the same, they're essentially two different diseases.

The inflammatory types of arthritis are autoimmune diseases and are related to a wide range of other autoimmune diseases in which the body's natural defense system turns on itself, including psoriasis, lupus, type 1 diabetes, celiac disease, and inflammatory bowel disease. The most common of these is rheumatoid arthritis, affecting 1.3 million Americans.

Osteoarthritis, also known as degenerative arthritis or wear-and-tear arthritis, is by far the more common type, with more than fifty million adults in the United States reporting being told by a doctor that they have some symptom of the disease. This does not include the millions of people who have the disease without any current symptoms. Yes, many if not most people with osteoarthritis have the disease for many years before symptoms appear.

Aging and Arthritis

A common myth that needs to be debunked is that aging is the primary cause of arthritis. No doubt there is a correlation between age and arthritis, but increasingly we know that age is not the cause. We'll explore the current science on why we get arthritis in the next chapter, but we've known for a long time now that osteoarthritis can arise either directly or indirectly. Simple wear and tear of the joints over time is an example of a direct cause. Another is that some individuals appear to be genetically predisposed, but this link has yet to be specifically established.

The secondary or indirect form of osteoarthritis results from a previous trauma to a joint, such as a fracture or a dislocation. This traumatic event sets off a reaction that can slowly increase the destruction of the joint over time. As a professor of orthopedic surgery and a sports medicine specialist, I see a multitude of young athletes, and I can predict which ones are likely to suffer from osteoarthritis later in life because of their sports injuries; often these individuals will begin to have symptoms in their late thirties. But now, because they are young and feel invincible, they will continue to overuse these injured joints, and sooner rather than later the joints will become arthritic.

Common Symptoms

While the term *arthritis* describes many diseases, they share common symptoms. Patients experience pain and stiffness in the joint early in the morning when they get out of bed. Often during the course of the day, when joints are being used a lot, or when patients have been on their feet for long periods of time, symptoms can increase. If patients slow down and rest, such as when sitting in a car or a chair, the stiffness will recur when they begin moving again.

Patients may experience fatigue due to the ongoing symptoms, and emotional stress can certainly become a major part of their lives. Some forms of arthritis can cause fevers, weight loss, and involvement of other organs, including kidneys, heart, and lungs. Rashes have also been seen with some forms of inflammatory arthritis.

Loss of the ability to work and to pursue recreational interests can exacerbate the stress associated with arthritis. In my practice, emotional reactions and depression are the most common psychological symptoms I see in my patients. I believe that this is most often a result of physical limitations and suffering. My patient Mrs. Dodd complained that her symptoms limited daily activities such as walking and doing household chores. Her depression and disturbed sleep also contributed to her disability and diminished her quality of life.

Common Types of Inflammatory Arthritis

While much of the rest of the book is devoted to osteoarthritis, this section discusses inflammatory forms of arthritis. These tend to be seen more often in younger people, and there are also gender differences, with women more prone to getting rheumatoid arthritis and lupus, while men are more prone to ankylosing spondylitis and gout. Some types of inflammatory arthritis, such as rheumatoid arthritis, can be intermittent, with remissions and flare-ups; in these cases, symptoms can often be controlled with medications. Long-lasting, chronic forms of any arthritis usually can be controlled with activity modification, protection of joints, exercise, medication, and patient education. Though we cannot make the disease go away, patients certainly can learn to live within the physical restrictions of the disease.

Rheumatoid Arthritis

Rheumatoid arthritis (RA) is an inflammation of the synovium, the tissue that lines the inside of a joint. In RA, the immune system becomes engaged and sends white blood cells to the joints as though there were an infection. This immune response is considered an autoimmune disease, as it seems the body attacks its own tissues as if they were foreign bodies. Diagnosis is by a blood test that measures rheumatoid factor, which will reveal if the disease is rheumatoid or another type of arthritis. No one knows the exact cause of rheumatoid arthritis, and as molecular biology techniques continue to evolve we continue to define different subsets of rheumatoid arthritis.

The reaction of the synovium membrane to RA is one of thickening, swelling, and proliferation of the cells. Over a period of time, this inflamed tissue continues to grow and produce proteins that eventually damage the articular cartilage and the bone of the joint. The joint can no longer move easily, and it enters a vicious cycle of swelling and inflammation.

Along with severe pain, RA can cause deformity. We know that heredity can increase your chances of having RA, but we do not know what causes the disease. RA crosses all racial, ethnic, and age categories, but women are two to three times more likely than men to have this disease.

RA usually begins in one or two joints and then can spread to many joints in the body. Most commonly affected are the fingers, hands, wrists, elbows, shoulders, knees, ankles, and feet; usually the involvement is symmetrical from left to right. Even the spine can be involved.

Arthritic joints are swollen and warm to the touch because of the increased blood supply that the inflammation brings. Occasional episodes of increased pain can occur; these are considered a "flare" of the disease. Flares can be related to stress or even changes in the weather, especially in increasingly cold temperatures. When pain decreases, either temporarily or permanently, it is known as remission. Flare-ups and remissions can come and go.

Patients with RA complain of stiffness of the joints, especially morning stiffness. Patients also may fatigue easily. Occasionally, lumps of firm tissue, known as rheumatoid nodules, can form underneath the skin. They can become irritated, especially when they are located near the elbow, as we tend to rest on our elbows when we're sitting or lying.

RA is usually a chronic, lifelong disease. It is difficult to predict how individuals will do over the course of this disease, as diagnosis is not always an exact science. A combination of medical history, physical exam, and several different blood and laboratory tests can help with a definitive diagnosis.

Treatment for this disease usually involves nonsteroidal anti-inflammatory drugs (NSAIDs) such as aspirin and ibuprofen. Activity modifications can help painful joints. Surgery (partial or total joint replacement) can also alleviate an advanced form of the disease in which joints have been destroyed. Other drugs that intervene in different aspects of the disease process, including new biologic drugs such as Enbrel (etanercept) and Humira (adalimumab), can help manage inflammation. Although RA can be progressive and painful, overall patients can lead normal, productive lives.

Systemic Lupus Erythematosus

Systemic lupus erythematosus (SLE) is also categorized as an autoimmune disease, as the body's immune system mistakenly attacks healthy tissue. This leads to long-term inflammation. It is diagnosed with a screening blood test.

SLE is much more common in women than in men. It may occur at any age but appears most often in people between the ages of ten and fifty. African Americans and Asians are affected more often than people of other races.

Symptoms vary from person to person and may come and go. Almost everyone with SLE has joint pain and swelling. Some develop arthritis. Frequently affected joints are the fingers, hands, wrists, and knees. Other common symptoms of SLE include chest pain when taking a deep breath, fatigue, fever with no other cause, general discomfort, uneasiness or ill feeling (malaise), hair loss, mouth sores, sensitivity to sunlight, skin rash, a "butterfly" rash over the cheeks and bridge of the nose, and swollen lymph nodes.

Depending on what part of the body is affected, additional symptoms can occur. For example, if the brain and nervous system are involved, the patient may have headaches, numbness, tingling, seizures, vision problems, or personality changes. If it is the digestive tract, the person may experience abdominal pain, nausea, and vomiting. When the heart is affected, the result may be abnormal heart rhythms. Symptoms from lung involvement can include coughing up blood and difficulty breathing. When the skin is involved its color may turn patchy and fingers may change color when cold.

Treatments include high-dose corticosteroids, to decrease the immune system response, or cytotoxic drugs, which block cell growth. As these medications can have serious side effects, you should be closely monitored by your doctor.

Progressive Systemic Sclerosis (PSS or Scleroderma)

One of the names of this rare form of inflammatory arthritis, scleroderma, derives from the Greek *sclero,* meaning "hard," and *derma,* "skin." The characteristic sign of this disease is thick, rigid skin on the arms and the face. Diagnosis is by blood testing.

PSS may affect many areas of the body, including joints, skin, heart, kidneys, intestinal tract, and lungs. Though this disease can affect people of any age and sex, most commonly it is seen in women between thirty and fifty years of age.

Diagnosis of PSS is difficult. Changes in the skin of the fingers, hands, and face such as widening of capillaries or calcium deposits are very typical of this disease as it advances. Patients may also display Raynaud's phenomenon—cold sensitivity that affects especially the fingers and toes. Many people with PSS have difficulty swallowing due to abnormal functioning of the esophagus.

Treatment consists of anti-inflammatory drugs, though corticosteroids are used when there are severe inflammatory problems. Overall, the prognosis for patients with PSS has improved over the years, and they generally can live productive, normal lives if they carefully watch for any other organ involvement.

Ankylosing Spondylitis (AS)

This chronic inflammatory disease affects joints in the spinal area, including the joints of the pelvic bones, the sacroiliac joints, and the spine itself. There is inflammation where the tendons and ligaments attach to bones (a condition known as enthesopathy). These inflammatory changes can lead to excessive bone formation in this area and fusing of the spine, resulting in stiffness and an inability to bend. There is no single blood test to diagnose AS.

This disease generally affects young men in their twenties and thirties. Early symptoms of the disease are morning stiffness and pain in the lower spine, especially around the sacroiliac joints. Patients may have arthritis in other joints as well as other symptoms such as fatigue and weight loss.

Treatment is generally with nonsteroidal anti-inflammatory drugs and physical therapy to maintain as much spine and joint flexibility as possible. Most patients have mild to moderate symptoms and lead normal, productive lives.

Gout and Pseudogout

Gout, one of the most intensely painful types of arthritis, accounts for 5 percent of all cases of arthritis, affecting about 5.1 million adults. Pain, inflammation, swelling, warmth, and redness of a single joint are typical symptoms. The big toe is the joint most commonly affected, but other joints can also be involved. Anyone can develop gout, but more men than women are affected by the disease. Those at greatest risk are men over the age of forty and women past menopause.

Gout is caused by the accumulation of excess uric acid in the body, resulting in the formation of crystals. The deposition of these crystals in the joints causes the inflammatory response.

Pseudogout is a condition that is often mistaken for gout. However, a different crystal, calcium pyrophosphate, is responsible for pseudo-gout. The knees are most commonly affected, but wrists, shoulders, ankles, elbows, or hands can also be affected.

The symptoms of gout and pseudogout can be misleading, as they resemble those seen in other types of inflammatory arthritis. A proper diagnosis comes from identifying the crystal in the fluid of the affected joint. In gout, the crystals may also be found as deposits under the skin, called tophi (pl.; sing., *tophus*).

Gout is typically treated with diet modification, as the body produces uric acid when it breaks down purines, substances that are found in many of the protein-rich foods we eat. Additional treatment includes weight reduction, adequate fluid intake, and the use of medications that control the inflammation, such as NSAIDs or corticosteroids. Other gout medications include colchicine, for acute gout attacks; allopurinol, which stops production of uric acid; and probenecid, which helps with elimination of uric acid. There are new drugs coming to market that promise to block inflammation reactions with a single injection.

Pseudogout is treated using anti-inflammatory drugs and low doses of colchicine.

Juvenile Rheumatoid Arthritis (JRA)

This type of arthritis affects two hundred thousand children in the United States. Generally, females are more affected than males, and usually sufferers are under sixteen years old. The specific cause of this disease is unknown.

JRA is similar to rheumatoid arthritis, although the symptoms in children are not the same as in adults. There are three types of JRA: one form affects the joints, one form affects the spine, and the third type is characterized by high fevers. Symptoms vary but often involve fever, weakness, anemia, and generalized joint pain and stiffness.

Treatment is with NSAIDs and physical therapy to prevent tightness of the joints. Diagnosis is difficult but is based on a combination of history, physical exam, and blood tests. Fortunately, most children outgrow this disease over time and do not have any long-term problems.

Polymyositis

Polymyositis is a rare disease that generally affects larger muscles located close to the body, such as the shoulders, upper arms, hips, and thighs. When these muscles become inflamed, they can become painful and weak. More women have this disease than men, and it generally involves people over thirty years of age.

Symptoms usually come on gradually, with weakness generally being the first symptom, evidenced by difficulty getting out of a chair or out of bed in the morning. Occasionally the skin can be affected with a rash.

This is a systemic disease, like RA, and it can include other symptoms, such as generalized weakness, weight loss, fevers, and Raynaud's phenomenon (an extreme sensitivity to cold, especially in the fingers and toes). The cause of this disease is uncertain. Treatment is with corticosteroids, which can reduce inflammation and increase muscle strength. Most patients respond well and lead normal, active lifestyles.

Polymyalgia Rheumatica

Severe stiffness about the neck, hips, and shoulders is known as polymyalgia rheumatica and is usually self-limiting. The symptoms generally occur in people over fifty, affecting more women than men. This disease is difficult to diagnose, as there is really no specific test and diagnosis is based on exams, medical history, and a series of negative test results.

Fibromyalgia

Although it's commonly thought of as an immune disease, fibromyalgia is not really one. Fibromyalgia is characterized by widespread musculo-skeletal pain accompanied by fatigue and problems with sleep, memory, and mood. The pain associated with fibromyalgia often is described as a constant dull ache in the muscles, with additional pain when firm pressure is applied to specific areas of the body, called tender points. Tender point locations include the back of the head, the front of the neck, between the shoulder blades and the top of the shoulders, the upper chest, the outer elbows, the upper part and sides of the hips, and the inner part of the knees. Researchers believe that fibromyalgia amplifies painful sensations by affecting the way the brain processes pain signals.

In some people symptoms begin after a physical trauma, surgery, infection, or significant psychological stress. Post-traumatic stress disorder has been linked to fibromyalgia. In others, symptoms gradually accumulate over time with no single triggering event. Because fibromyalgia tends to run in families, there may be certain genetic mutations that make you more susceptible to developing the disorder. Some illnesses appear to trigger or aggravate fibromyalgia. Women are much more likely to develop fibromyalgia than are men.

Many patients who have fibromyalgia also have tension headaches, temporomandibular joint (TMJ) disorders, irritable bowel syndrome, anxiety, and depression. Often sufferers of the disease tend to awaken tired, as sleep is often disrupted by pain. It is frequently accompanied by other sleep disorders such as sleep apnea and restless leg syndrome, further worsening symptoms.

While there is no cure for fibromyalgia, a variety of medications can help control symptoms. Exercise, relaxation, and stress reduction measures also have been known to relieve associated joint inflammation.

Bursitis and Tendinitis

Bursitis and tendinitis are both common conditions that involve inflammation of the soft tissue around muscles and bones, most often in the shoulder, elbow, wrist, hip, knee, or ankle. Carpenters, gardeners, musicians, athletes, and others who perform activities that require repetitive motions or place stress on joints are at higher risk for tendinitis and bursitis. An infection, arthritis, gout, thyroid disease, and diabetes can also bring about bursitis or tendinitis.

Tendinitis is inflammation or irritation of a tendon, the thick, fibrous cords that attach muscles to bone. Tendons transmit the power generated by a muscle contraction to move a bone. They are found throughout the body, including the hands, wrists, elbows, shoulders, hips, knees, ankles, and feet. Tendons can be small, like those found in the hand, or large, like the Achilles tendon in the heel.

Tendinitis is most often the result of a repetitive injury or motion in the affected area. For example, rotator cuff injuries are associated with the throwing motion found in certain sports, and tennis elbow is inflammation associated with a partial tear of the tendon. These conditions occur more often in older individuals, as tendons become less flexible with age and therefore more prone to injury.

Bursitis occurs when a bursa becomes inflamed. A bursa is a small, fluid-filled sac that acts as a cushion between a bone and other moving parts, such as muscles, tendons, or skin. Bursitis is commonly caused by overuse or direct trauma to a joint and often occurs at the knee or elbow; it can be caused by kneeling on a hard surface or leaning on the elbows longer than usual, for example. Shoulder bursitis is very common with hand use in the overhead position.

Since both tendons and bursae are located near joints, inflammation in these soft tissues will often be perceived by patients as joint pain and mistaken for osteoarthritis. Symptoms of bursitis and tendinitis are similar: pain and stiffness aggravated by movement. Pain may be prominent at night. Almost any tendon or bursa in the body can be affected, but those located around a joint are most often involved. Tendinitis and bursitis are usually temporary conditions but may become chronic problems. Unlike arthritis, they do not cause deformity, but they can limit motion.

Treatment of tendinitis and bursitis is based on the underlying cause. In overuse or injury, reduction or avoidance of a particular activity is useful. Splinting the affected area, applying moist heat or sometimes ice, and using other forms of physical therapy are helpful. Anti-inflammatory medications can reduce inflammation and pain. Corticosteroid injections into the affected area are frequently helpful. If an infection is present, an appropriate antibiotic is necessary and serial aspiration or surgical intervention, although uncommon, may be required.

Once the acute attack of tendinitis or bursitis subsides, preventing recurrences is relatively easy. Proper conditioning, adequate warm-up, ergonomically correct workstations, proper joint positioning, and appropriate splints or pads to protect susceptible areas can all help to prevent recurrences.

Anatomy of a Joint

Understanding what a joint looks like, how joints function, and how arthritis develops will put you in a better position to know what you can do to help yourself.

Arthritis can affect any joint that has articular cartilage, including the hands, wrists, elbows, shoulders, knees, ankles, feet, hips, back, and neck. It can also affect the inside lining or synovium of the joint.

Inflammatory arthritis generally affects the hands, wrists, elbows, shoulders, knees, and ankles in different combinations. The weight-bearing joints, such as the knees, hips, and back, tend to incur more wear and tear and therefore are more commonly associated with osteoarthritis.

Types of Joints

There are three types of joints in the body. Fibrous joints occur when bones are held together in a way that does not permit any movement. For example, the bones of the skull come together in fibrous joints. Cartilaginous joints connect bones by means of cartilage only, which allows very little movement; this is the case with the ribs, for example. The third type of joint, synovial-lined joints, is the most relevant to a discussion of arthritis, because these joints are highly mobile and play an important part in the everyday motion of our limbs. They come in various shapes, including a ball and socket (hip), hinge (elbow), and saddle (knee), and different sizes. These free-moving joints are the ones most often disabled by arthritis.

Structure of the Human Synovial Joint

All synovial joints have a capsule that surrounds the ends of the bones. The inside of this capsule is lined with a thin tissue that produces fluid to lubricate the joint. On the top or side of the joint are muscles and tendons, which move the bones. Ligaments, which can be located inside or outside the joint, secure the ends of bones to each other, rigidly controlling each joint's specific individual range of motion.

Joint Capsule

The joint capsule consists of two layers of tissue. The outer layer is tough and fibrous, helping to hold the ends of bones together and prevent excessive movement of the bones. Inside the joint capsule is the synovium or synovial membrane, which produces fluid that both lubricates and nourishes the cartilage. Both of these layers of the joint capsule have a strong blood supply as well as many nerve endings.

Articular Cartilage

The human skeleton consists of more than three hundred bones that provide a rigid framework to protect the organs and allow motion through muscle contraction. Specific bones are connected by approximately 150 joints, which allow motion in confined muscular planes. The ends of a bone are covered with a shock-absorbing tissue called articular hyaline cartilage. This articular cartilage is very slippery and smooth, providing easy motion at the ends of the bones. It is almost a frictionless environment, which helps joints function through a lifetime of repetitive use.

Articular cartilage consists of a structure of intertwined strands of complex proteins, collagen and proteoglycans, surrounded by water.

Collagen is a gelatinous, fibrous substance that can be compressed and springs back into shape once the pressure is released (something you can see when you bend your ears, which are largely made up of cartilage). The collagen in the cartilage gives the joint its shock-absorbing abilities.

Special cartilage-forming cells, known as chondrocytes, are located throughout the articular cartilage. These chondrocytes manufacture and maintain the cartilage's collagen and proteoglycans.

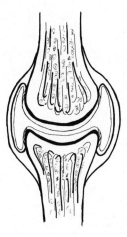

FIGURE 1. Schematic diagram of a normal joint with smooth articular cartilage covering bone.

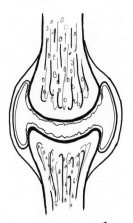

FIGURE 2. Schematic diagram of an osteoarthritic joint with degenerating articular cartilage.

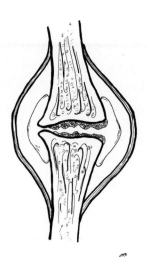

FIGURE 3. Advancing osteoarthritis with increasing cartilage degeneration and synovium thickening.

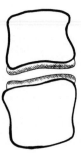 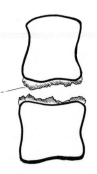

FIGURE 4. Schematic drawing of a vertebral body of the spine with and without articular cartilage degeneration.

The Arthritis Process

Unlike some diseases that occur and then resolve completely, arthritis gets progressively worse as cartilage continues to degrade and joints and bones are damaged.

Cartilage Degeneration

The most common form of arthritis, osteoarthritis, is caused by wearing away of the cartilage that cushions the ends of the bones. Under normal conditions, the chondrocytes in the articular cartilage continually replenish the cartilage's collagen and proteoglycans. But because the chondrocytes do not have a good blood supply, when they are damaged they do not heal easily, and over time not enough new cartilage is generated by the remaining healthy chondrocytes to replace what has been worn away. The chondrocytes can be damaged by either biomechanical or biochemical changes in the joint.

As cartilage degrades, its smooth surface can develop cracks and holes. Over time the bone underneath the cartilage can be exposed. One consequence may be the formation of cysts. Another consequence may be the development of bony spurs, which are thought to be part of the body's response to help stabilize and repair the joint. The joint frequently becomes enlarged, sometimes visibly so (this is often seen in finger joints).

When the cartilage has eroded sufficiently, bone begins to rub on bone, causing pain and further wear and tear. This process creates inflammation, swelling, and sometimes redness. Particles from broken-down tissue cause further chemical inflammation. Generally, there is increased pain and stiffness, with decreased joint motion. These symptoms progressively worsen, especially if the joint is used repetitively. However, in osteoarthritis synovial inflammation is seldom as severe as in rheumatoid arthritis.

Synovitis

Synovitis, an inflammation of the joint lining, is the classic process seen in inflammatory arthritis. With synovitis, the normally smooth, thin synovial inner membrane becomes thickened and the fluid within the joint becomes more viscous because of all the white blood cells it contains. These cells and the chemical reactions they are involved in can wear away bone and cartilage. The tendons and ligaments around the joint can also be weakened, either by the inflammatory process or by the damage to the joint. Drug treatment can slow this inflammatory process.

Takeaways

Arthritis isn't just one disease but a hundred or more different diseases, many of which are associated with an autoimmune dysfunction in which the body's own defense mechanisms inadvertently attack and inflame the joints. On the other hand, osteoarthritis, which is far more common, is the result of wear and tear (although in the next chapter we'll see how increasingly it's thought that inflammation plays a leading role in the cause, too). Blood and other diagnostic tests can determine what type of arthritis you have.

2

WHY WE GET ARTHRITIS

To understand current thinking about the causes of osteoarthritis, you have to know why Kobe Bryant left for Germany immediately after the Los Angeles Lakers lost in the 2012 NBA playoffs against the Oklahoma City Thunder. It's not that the team's captain had a particular fondness for Dusseldorf, his destination in Germany—the city is hardly anyone's idea of a vacation paradise.

Rather, the thirty-four-year-old basketball superstar was headed for a medical clinic he'd been to many times during the off season to treat his arthritic knee with an experimental process called Regenokine. (The reason he travels to Germany to get Regenokine is that it's not FDA-approved for use in the United States, although off-label treatments are being given here.)

The treatment is similar to another therapy called PRP, both of which involve isolating a patient's blood platelets and other growth factors and reinjecting them into the damaged body part (in Bryant's case, his arthritic knee). We'll dig deeper into the science of Regenokine, PRP, and other next-generation biologic treatments later in the book. For now, it's enough to know that all these treatments aim to accelerate the body's natural healing process by stopping one thing: inflammation.

When Inflammation Was Just a Symptom

From a clinical perspective, pain relief is an important part of treatment. But the exciting stuff in research is figuring out how to stop inflammation.

Why is inflammation so important? Ten or fifteen years ago, most orthopedic surgeons and clinicians would have looked at inflammation as a *symptom* of osteoarthritis (OA). The cartilage deteriorates over time or through trauma (like Kobe Bryant's repeated knee injuries). Joints lose their protective cushioning, bones grind together, and the surrounding tissue swells and becomes inflamed. It made perfect sense—that is, if you didn't scratch beneath the surface and start asking exactly why the cartilage begins to deteriorate. The correlation between age and cartilage degradation didn't mean there was a causal relationship between the two.

The conventional wisdom about inflammation and arthritis took a big hit beginning in the early 2000s. About that time a number of medical researchers in different disciplines starting thinking that inflammation was the common factor in all chronic diseases, including arthritis, and that figuring out how to control inflammation was the key to unlocking the cure. At first such theories were the stuff of esoteric biomedical journals. But by 2004 the theory had entered popular culture, and it even made the cover of *Time* magazine on February 24 that year, with the headline "The Secret Killer: The Surprising Link Between Inflammation and Heart Attacks, Cancer, Alzheimer's and Other Diseases." The article began intriguingly:

> What does a stubbed toe or a splinter in a finger have to do with your risk of developing Alzheimer's disease, suffering a heart attack or succumbing to colon cancer? More than you might think. As scientists delve deeper into the fundamental causes of those and other illnesses, they are starting to see links to an age-old immunological defense mechanism called inflammation—the same biological process that turns the tissue around a splinter red and causes swelling in an injured toe. If they are right—and the evidence is starting to look pretty good—it could radically change doctors' concept of what makes us sick.

Welcome but Unintended Consequences

One of the "other diseases" mentioned on the *Time* cover may have been what got the whole inflammation-as-cause theory rolling. In 1999, Celebrex (celecoxib), a new type of prescription drug from pharmaceutical giant Pfizer, was introduced to the public. Like other nonsteroidal anti-inflammatory drugs, Celebrex promised to inhibit the body's inflammation process—with less of the gastrointestinal irritation associated with NSAIDs.

Celebrex became the best-selling drug launch in history—a testimony in large part to the increasing ranks of arthritis sufferers. Today, Celebrex continues to garner huge profits, grossing more than $3.1 billion in sales in 2011.

Shortly after the drug's release, an unintended but welcome consequence appeared. Researchers noticed that patients who took the drug were less likely to develop intestinal polyps—abnormal growths that can become cancerous. If the correlation held up, it might indicate that the anti-inflammatory effects of the drug—designed to stop pain—were also decreasing the risk of cancer.

About the same time, cardiologists discovered that the new group of cholesterol-lowering drugs called statins were far more effective at preventing heart attacks than anyone had expected. It turns out that statins don't just lower cholesterol levels; they also reduce inflammation. (Today statins are being tested for possible effectiveness in Alzheimer's disease and sickle-cell anemia as well.)

This new view of inflammation changed how scientists did medical research. Suddenly, in medical schools and research institutions across the United States, cardiologists, rheumatologists, oncologists, allergists, and neurologists began comparing notes—and realized that they were looking at inflammation as an explanation for just about everything having to do with chronic disease.

To understand how revolutionary this idea was, it's useful to explore how most doctors viewed heart disease until recently. (Funding spent on heart disease research dwarfs that spent on arthritis. While far more people are affected by arthritis, heart disease remains the number one killer of Americans, which is why it gets the big research money.) Until recently, heart disease was viewed as a "plumbing problem" of clogged arteries. Over the years, fatty deposits would slowly build up on the insides of major coronary arteries until they grew so big that they cut off the supply of blood to a vital part of the heart. A complex molecule called LDL, the so-called bad cholesterol, provided the raw material for these deposits. The higher your LDL levels, the greater your chance for clogged arteries and your risk of heart attack.

There's just one problem with this theory: half of all heart attacks occur in people with normal cholesterol levels. Not only that, but as imaging techniques improved, doctors found, again much to their surprise, that the most dangerous plaques weren't necessarily all that large. Something that hadn't yet been identified was causing those deposits to burst, triggering massive clots that cut off the coronary blood supply. Again, all fingers pointed to inflammation.

Inflammation Cause and Effect

But let's back up even further for a moment. Now we're learning that inflammation is probably the underlying cause of a wide range of chronic diseases, including arthritis. But why does inflammation occur in the first place?

Inflammation is a key tool of the body's immune system. If you cut yourself, the body sends in a barrage of microbe-fighting chemicals, including one called histamine, as a first-line defense to search out and then attack any bacteria attempting to slip into the wound. The histamine and other chemicals cause the nearby capillaries to leak, allowing plasma to enter the fray; this slows down the foreign invaders and paves the way for more powerful immune defenders—the cavalry, if you will—to join the battle. As the capillaries expand, the wound becomes red, hot, and swollen. When the threat of infection recedes, so does the inflammation.

But it isn't the temporary inflammation associated with cuts, bruises, and other trauma that's the problem. Rather, the real culprit is the long-term variety that results from cigarette smoke, excess cholesterol, and barely detectable but lingering infections. The resulting low-grade, chronic inflammation is what's thought to be associated with chronic disease.

The next step was the hypothesis that inflammation could not only result from but actually cause the loss of cartilage that is the main symptom of osteoarthritis. It seemed counterintuitive and flew in the face of what was believed to be true about arthritis: that the body's cartilage wears down with age—just like tires on a car—and that's that.

Here's to You, Mr. Robinson

Stanford immunologist Bill Robinson, MD, PhD, and his colleagues challenged that timeworn truism, showing in a 2011 study how an initial insult, such as a torn meniscus (a crescent-shaped piece of cartilage-rich tissue that helps cushion the knee), could trigger a cascade of low-grade inflammatory activity in the joint that could in turn result in the cartilage destruction that is osteoarthritis—sometimes years after the injury.

The so-called complement cascade that Robinson identified in osteoarthritis is a complex and multifaceted phenomenon. It appears that the cascade can damage cartilage at various stages—sometimes stopping at one stage while at other times proceeding to a far more advanced condition.

And it's not just trauma that triggers the cascade. Bacterial and viral infections can cause the chronic inflammation chain reaction to begin. Upon activation of the complement cascade, these proteins engage in a complex interplay, culminating in the activation of a protein cluster called MAC (membrane attack complex). By punching holes in the membranes of human cells infected with a bacterium or a virus, MAC helps to clear the body of infection.

The new study showed that, indeed, initial damage to the joint—from trauma or infection—sets in motion a chain of molecular events that escalates into an attack upon the damaged joint by one of the body's key defense systems against bacterial and viral infections, the complement system.

An early clue regarding the complement system's key role in osteoarthritis came when Robinson and his colleagues compared the levels of large numbers of proteins present in the joint fluid taken from osteoarthritis patients with levels present in fluid from healthy individuals. They found that the patients' tissues had a relative overabundance of proteins that act as accelerators in the complement cascade, along with a dearth of proteins that act as brakes on this cascade.

Robinson's group also examined the activity level of joint-lining tissues of osteoarthritic subjects versus those of healthy subjects and observed a similar result: in the arthritis patients there was more expression of genes encoding complement-activating and related inflammatory proteins, and less expression of genes encoding complement- and inflammation-inhibiting ones. (More on this in a moment.)

Of Mice and Meniscus

The researchers decided to see if they could use their newly gained knowledge of the complement cascade to actually induce or prevent osteoarthritis in laboratory mice. They induced the equivalent of meniscal tears in mice who (like humans) are much more prone to getting osteoarthritis in joints that have suffered such damage. In humans, the meniscus is the bane of runners, as it seems prone to tearing after long runs. Meniscal tears also can appear spontaneously as one grows older. In fact, about one in five people ages fifty to fifty-nine, and more than half of people over seventy, have experienced one. The experimental procedure was performed on normal mice and on three separate strains of bioengineered lab mice, each strain missing a different protein component of the complement system. In two cases, the missing protein was one that ordinarily acts as an accelerator within the complement cascade, and in the third case the one that was missing usually acts as a brake.

The normal mice developed osteoarthritis, as expected. But the two strains of bioengineered mice lacking the protein that would accelerate the inflammation cascade developed less-severe arthritis than the normal mice, while the mice lacking the protein that would normally brake the cascade got worse faster.

Next, Robinson's team tried to figure out how the complement cascade was causing osteoarthritis. Further experiments in mice and with human tissue showed that MAC, the membrane-busting heavy artillery of the system, was damaging the cells in joint tissue—but not by punching holes in them. Instead, it was binding to cartilage-producing cells in these tissues and causing them to secrete still more cascade-inducing proteins as well as other inflammatory chemicals. Specialized enzymes that chewed up and spat out cartilage also were getting into the act.

What they found, ultimately, was that a continuing cycle of joint-tissue damage—not trauma (the meniscal tears)—induced osteoarthritis. Now that a specific inflammatory pathway had been identified in the development of osteoarthritis, suddenly it was beginning to look like a real disease, not just a collective term for degenerating cartilage and aching joints.

Understanding the cause of the disease is the first step in finding a possible cure for osteoarthritis. By implicating the complement cascade, in the initiation of osteoarthritis, Robinson and his colleagues pointed to a new target for drugs that could pull the rug out from under osteoarthritis before it started.

A Cure? It's Complicated

Now that we know inflammation is likely a primary, foundational cause of OA, why don't we do something about it?

If the key is taming the body's immune system so it doesn't attack the body's tissues with an under-the-radar, persistent inflammation, then there are three ways to go about it, as an article in *Newsweek* succinctly put it: "You can reduce the triggers that cause inflammation. You can hamper the cellular 'master switches' that orchestrate the body's inflammatory response. Or you can knock out the inflammatory chemicals," the substances that actually produce the inflammation.

Here's the catch. If you turn down the various components of the immune system, you run the risk of pathogens entering the body unfettered. Oncologists deliberately turn down the immune system when treating cancer with chemotherapy—they flood the body with toxins that kill the cancerous cell but fell a good deal of the immune cells at the same time. In cancer patients, the temporary damage to the immune system can be compensated for by powerful antibiotics that will knock out any disease-causing microbes that enter the patient's body. But for chronic inflammation, that's not a sustainable solution, because antibiotics cause their own problems.

A few years ago a very promising drug called Tysabri (natalizumab) was developed to treat multiple sclerosis, a devastating autoimmune disease that often surfaces in young adulthood, just as its sufferers are beginning their families. The drug was designed to modulate the immune system, in effect halting it from systematically attacking its host body. But several patients taking it with another medication called Avonex developed an additional neurodegenerative disease, this one caused by a latent virus that most of us harbor.

Beyond Chronic Inflammation

It wasn't too many years ago that understanding free radicals (chemically unstable molecules) and the oxidative damage they caused to cellular structure was considered the key to unlocking chronic disease—that is, before inflammation seized the limelight. Neuroscientist James Joseph of Tufts University has quipped that "inflammation is the evil twin of oxidation. Where you find one, you find the other."

To be sure, the free radical camp has not given up on finding a cure for osteoarthritis by addressing oxidative damage. Some researchers, for example, are looking at how nitrous oxide, a highly reactive free radical implicated in tissue injury in a variety of diseases, might play a key role in cartilage degradation. Cartilage obtained from patients with osteoarthritis produces excess nitrous oxide. Could the inhibition of nitrous oxide be a key to future therapeutic strategies?

Other researchers are looking at the component parts of the inflammation cascade. For example, interleukin-1 beta (IL-1B) is probably one of the most powerful of these inflammatory factors when it comes to the destructive process in joints. IL-1B is part of a group of substances called cytokines, which are signaling molecules used extensively in cellular communication and in particular are secreted by immune cells when they encounter a pathogen. IL-1B prevents the formation of new, healthy chondrocytes by promoting inflammation, thus preventing adequate renewal of cartilage. At the same time, IL-1B produces proteases, which are enzymes that break down proteins. In the case of osteoarthritis, proteases contribute to the destructive process.

The inflammation cascade is really a complicated series of chemical reactions involving numerous factors: cytokines, enzymes, peptides, and amino acids, to name just a few. One of the signaling cascades that has been identified in osteoarthritic destruction is the activation of a protein called NF-kB. This protein moves into the cell nucleus and starts talking with various regulatory genes. These regulatory genes decide when cells die (a process called apoptosis), when inflammatory cells are activated, and when other immune responses are initiated. NF-kB actually regulates at least 150 genes, some of which are directly involved with inflammation and immune function.

Through studies of families, we know that genetic factors are implicated in some way in the development of osteoarthritis, though we don't know precisely which ones or how they operate. If scientists can discover the precise genes involved and figure out how to turn them off (or on, as the case may be), then they may be on the path to controlling or even preventing the disease.

Gene Expression and Red Grapes

Since we've introduced the topic of genes and osteoarthritis, let's look at another one that's of interest to osteoarthritis researchers: SIRT-1.

If you Google "SIRT-1," you're likely to come across websites mentioning the putative life-extending value of a protein produced by this gene. One site even has close-up photos comparing monkeys who more effectively express the SIRT-1 gene with monkeys of the same age who have "bad" expression of the gene. In comparison, the ones with "good" expression of the gene look like Hollywood celebrities after an especially good face-lift. These websites are usually linked to a sales pitch for resveratrol, a natural substance produced by some plants (notably red grapes) that may be linked to activation of the SIRT-1 gene. We'll review the effectiveness of resveratrol and other over-the-counter supplements in Chapter 4. However, suffice it to say here that SIRT-1 is strongly linked to cell survival and proliferation.

Research has implicated SIRT-1 as a key factor in aging-related diseases, including osteoarthritis. In one recent study, cartilage samples from patients undergoing knee orthopedic surgery were examined. In severely degenerated cartilage, the protein produced by SIRT-1 was barely detectable. The conclusion is that the reduction of this protein in cartilage cells may cause them to self-destruct and may stiffen the normally flexible cellular matrix.

The AGEs Theory of Aging

Speaking of aging, we can't finish a discussion of theories about the cause of osteoarthritis without mentioning the AGEs theory. *AGEs* stands for "advanced glycation end products," substances that have been shown to be involved in various aspects of aging.

AGEs are proteins that have been damaged by carbohydrates that attach themselves to the proteins. As we grow older, AGEs accumulate in our tissues. It appears that AGEs released from affected tissue can migrate to the synovium around the joints, degrading the cartilage there. You can actually see the damage AGEs cause to cartilage: articular cartilage is normally bluish white and flexible, but articular cartilage affected by AGEs looks yellowish and is stiff.

Not All Fats Are Created Equal

When considering causes of osteoarthritis, one of them is all around us—namely, obesity. For many years now doctors have observed that patients who are clinically obese are at increased risk for osteoarthritis. Initially it was thought that this was a biomechanical effect—you try carrying an extra hundred pounds around with you 24/7 and see what your knees look like in ten years.

But researchers eventually began to realize that obese patients had osteoarthritis in their hands as well as in the load-bearing joints of the hips, ankles, and knees. At around the same time, other research was beginning to show that not all types of body fat were created equal. Once thought of as an inert substance devoted to energy storage, fat suddenly seemed to have a variety of effects in the body.

Accumulating evidence suggested that obesity causes low-grade inflammation—a systemic metabolic breakdown in which fat, particularly abdominal fat, functions as a quasi-living, breathing organ releasing bioactive substances called adipokines. These adipokines are pernicious, causing a reduced sensitivity to insulin that in turn can lead to metabolic syndrome and an increased risk of both type 2 diabetes and cardiovascular disease. *Diabesity*—a term linking obesity and diabetes—has now become a medical buzzword.

Moreover, studies of different adipokines reveal that they play pro-inflammatory and other biochemical roles in the development of osteoarthritis. In short: while being obese will increase the load on your joints, particularly your hips, knees, and ankles, if you carry most of your excess weight in your gut—the proverbial beer belly—then you're likely to have even more severe osteoarthritis in non-load-bearing joints such as those in the hands and neck.

Obesity has become such a bane for osteoarthritis patients and doctors such as me who try to treat them that the next chapter is entirely devoted to this new epidemic, which I call "obeseritis."

A Final Note on the Genesis of Osteoarthritis

As we've seen, the prevailing theory on the development of OA focuses on damage to joint cartilage. But a new theory was floated in 2013 by a team at Johns Hopkins University, who suggested that initial harm to the cartilage causes the bone underneath it to behave improperly, building surplus bone when it isn't needed. The extra bone stretches the cartilage above it and speeds its decline.

As one of the researchers, Xu Cao, noted, "If there is something wrong with the leg of your chair and you try to fix it by replacing the cushion, you haven't solved the problem." Added Cao, "We think that the problem in OA is not just the cartilage 'cushion,' but the bone underneath."

Could a treatment be developed, then, that focuses on stopping the growth of the surplus bone? The team has had success in the lab in blocking the bone-destruction process in mice. A clinical trial is being developed to test the same drug in humans. Stay tuned.

Takeaways

Let's summarize what we've learned. Once thought to be an affliction caused by the biomechanical wear and tear of the joints over time, osteoarthritis, we now know, is due in large degree to chronic inflammation. A cascade of overlapping factors likely causes the disease process—factors as diverse as bacterial and viral infections, free radicals and oxidative stress, gene expression, obesity, and metabolic syndrome.

Moving forward, the treatment of osteoarthritis will take into account all of this information and attempt to tailor treatments to how the disease manifests in a particular patient. Just as there are different kinds of arthritis and different causes for osteoarthritis, at last we've come to recognize there are different ways the disease appears in individual patients. It makes sense, doesn't it? Should we be treating a professional athlete in his prime such as Kobe Bryant in the same way as we would treat Mrs. Dodd, the elderly patient I discussed in Chapter 1? Of course not, but to date, that's how medicine has viewed osteoarthritis—one disease with one therapeutic strategy.

It's clear from all the overlapping findings about potential causes of osteoarthritis that before a cure can be found, scientists need much more detailed knowledge of how the various parts of the immune system interact. But we may be rapidly approaching the day when a blood test could tell us how to fine-tune treatment to each individual's immune system—allowing it to fight pathogens but also to avoid chronic inflammation.

In the chapters that follow we'll also discuss how researchers like me are taking a whole other tack, not worrying so much about the cause of osteoarthritis but rather focusing on replacing damaged cartilage with new cartilage generated from stem cells. But first, can we talk about your weight?

3

"OBESERITIS"

In the previous chapters we learned that if you live long enough, chances are you will eventually get arthritis. Let's recap the numbers:

- Fifty million adults in the United States are currently living with arthritis.

- Sixty to seventy million people are projected to be diagnosed with it by 2030.

- If you're currently fifty-five or older, you have a 75 percent chance of developing arthritis sometime during the rest of your life.

- By age seventy-nine, virtually everyone shows some arthritic symptoms.

- Thirty percent of those ages forty-five to sixty-nine have arthritis.

- Almost 8 percent of those ages eighteen to forty-four already have it.

The statistics become even more eye-opening when you figure into the picture the number of Americans who say they are hobbled by the disease. Over the last five years, there has been a significant jump in the percentage of adults who said their joint pain or other arthritis symptoms limited their usual activities, to 9.4 percent from 8.3 percent. This means that more than twenty-one million adults have trouble climbing stairs, dressing, gardening, or doing other things, according to researchers at the Centers for Disease Control (CDC).

Much of the problem occurs in our graying baby boomer population. More Americans are now at an age when they are likely to suffer from osteoarthritis, which breaks down cartilage and causes pain and joint stiffness.

But that doesn't explain the spike in reports of lack of mobility among arthritis sufferers. In other words, the typical arthritis sufferer is more debilitated than his or her counterpart twenty years ago. I can confirm this—I've seen it in my own practice over the past two decades. So what's going on here?

Just look around. We've become a nation of overweight people. Two-thirds of us are overweight, and 35 percent of Americans are now clinically obese. (Obesity is defined as being 20 percent or more over ideal body weight.) The rates are even higher for baby boomers. Think we're fat now? A new report from the Trust for America's Health predicts that if current trends continue, 44 percent of Americans will be obese by 2030. In the thirteen most affected states, 60 percent of residents will be obese in less than two decades.

What does fat have to do with arthritis? As we saw in Chapter 2, extra weight not only contributes to the biochemical causes of osteoarthritis but also puts more pressure on those arthritic joints, making the problem worse. The percentage of people who say their arthritis significantly affects their daily activities was more than twice as high among the obese as among those who were of normal weight or underweight, the CDC researchers found.

In another CDC study, the number of patients over age forty-five who visited the doctor at least once annually jumped by 26 percent during the past decade, while their actual portion of the population increased by only 11 percent. The researchers concluded that baby boomers and older Americans are seeing doctors more often to manage chronic conditions. Arthritis was the second most commonly seen of these conditions. Number one was high blood pressure, and in third place was diabetes—both of which, like arthritis, are obesity related.

Let's look at obesity in terms of its cost to society. One study found that obese patients in the United States incur 46 percent higher patient costs, have 27 percent more physician visits, and use 80 percent more prescription drugs than normal-weight people. The annual extra medical costs of obesity in the United States were estimated at more than $75 billion.

In the next two decades, if the trends we've seen since the early 1990s continue, obesity would result in 8 million more cases of diabetes, 6.8 million more cases of coronary heart disease and stroke, and an additional 500,000 cases of cancer. This will, of course, produce a huge expansion of obesity-related health care expenditure over the next two decades. Compounded by an aging population, obesity disorders will trigger a $28 billion increase in medical costs by 2020 and $66 billion by 2030.

Statistics aside, I can personally testify to the changing landscape. When I first began practicing medicine as an orthopedic surgery resident three decades ago, the typical arthritis sufferer was sixty years old and of normal weight. Today I'm seeing patients who are typically fifty-five years old and fifty pounds or more overweight. From a physician's perspective, the difference is shocking—and frustrating. The advances that we've made in the treatment of arthritis over the last two decades—medications, orthopedic devices, and physical therapy techniques—are being cannibalized by the excessive weight that the average arthritis patient now carries.

Indeed, obesity and arthritis have become so intertwined that it warrants a whole new term to describe this phenomenon: *obeseritis.*

Why Are We Getting Fatter?

The problem of obesity has become so serious that it's now thought of as a public health issue, just like the flu. And just like the flu, obesity knows no boundaries. Excess weight is rapidly becoming a major public health issue in developing countries as well as the industrialized world. It's now estimated that as much as 20 percent of the urbanized population in China is obese. Similar figures have been reported in India, with parts of major cities there reporting obesity rates topping 40 percent.

Obesity has become such a serious health concern that the editors of *Lancet,* one of the most influential medical journals in the world, recently published a series on obesity by some of the leading scientists in a wide array of fields that intersect with the topic, from health economics to nutrition and biomedical physiology. Their collective wisdom as to why the world is becoming fat? For the first time in history, advances in agricultural science and technology have made an abundance of cheap, easily accessed high-calorie food available to most of the people in the world. Combine that with an increasingly sedentary lifestyle for the human race, and the result is obesity. To look at it from a more physiological perspective, we're consuming too many calories in comparison to how much we expend.

How did we arrive at this juncture in medical history? The *Lancet* team has identified the tipping point, but first let me ask you a question: have you noticed how there are no fat people on the iconic TV series *Mad Men*? (Okay, Don Draper's second wife got heavy for one season, but that's because she was depressed.) The show has a reputation for being extraordinarily accurate in its depiction of life in the 1960s, from the clothes the characters wear to the furniture that surrounds them and the period jargon that they speak.

When it comes to weight, the producers of *Mad Men* were right again: the increased prevalence of obesity began in the 1970s despite the fact that most of the drivers of obesity were already in place by the 1960s, including an abundance of cheap food and a sedentary lifestyle abetted by mechanization and suburban sprawl (which discourages walking and promotes car travel). The *Lancet* team concluded that the difference between the two decades was that "the 1970s saw a striking rise in the quantity of refined carbohydrates and fats in the US food supply, which was paralleled by a sharp increase in available calories and the onset of the obesity epidemic." That is, the rise of junk food is threatening to overwhelm the health care system in the United States and, increasingly, everywhere else in the world.

Here's the great irony of the worldwide obesity epidemic: millions upon millions of people are starving from a lack of food at the same time. Some 1.46 billion people globally are considered overweight or "overnourished," but 1 billion people are suffering from undernourishment. Of the two problems, obesity has now tipped the scales, and according to the *Lancet* study, the "global burden of disease" has moved from undernourishment to overnourishment. To frame it another way, as recently as 1990 the leading cause of chronic disease worldwide was malnutrition; today it's obesity.

What Athletes Can Teach All of Us

But enough negativity! Here's the good news: you can decrease the symptoms of arthritis with easy-to-follow steps that really work. This program incorporates the same techniques I use with the athletes I see every week in my role as the chief of sports medicine at the Keck School of Medicine at the University of Southern California. What do college athletes have to do with baby boomers and arthritis? There are no fat athletes. With the exception of a few pro football linebackers and sumo wrestlers, fat doesn't work in competitive athletics.

Now, that doesn't mean athletes don't gain excess weight. But when they do, they get rid of it by using the irrefutable law of nature known as thermodynamics. Simply put, you gain weight when you consume more calories than you burn. Conversely, you lose weight when you consume fewer calories than you burn.

In this chapter, we'll demonstrate how a program of exercise—and not just any exercise, but a plan designed to tackle obesity *and* arthritis—combined with sensible diet can dramatically reduce the pain and immobility associated with osteoarthritis. This regimen of diet and exercise can be used as a foundation for anyone suffering from osteoarthritis, whether or not you're overweight.

In subsequent chapters, we'll put all the information together and then tailor it into a program specific to you, factoring in things such as your gender, fitness level, age, diet, race, medical history, occupation, and lifestyle.

Take Care of Thyself

All the advice in this chapter is oriented toward things you can do at home without the aid of a professional therapist or any fancy equipment. If you follow the steps in this chapter, you will reduce your chances of getting osteoarthritis; if you already have it, you can reduce your pain and increase your mobility.

However, before we get going, let me share with you my own arthritis story. While I wrote this book to give you the very latest, practical information for dealing with arthritis, I have to confess that I also wrote it for myself, a sixty-two-year-old white male who's maybe something of a workaholic—okay, I *am* a workaholic, typically putting in over sixty hours of work a week between my duties as a senior orthopedic surgeon at the Keck School of Medicine, my teaching responsibilities, and my own private practice and research endeavors. Yet I find time to work out at the gym, typically three times a week, and during the winter I pursue my lifelong passion for skiing as often as I can. And yes, I have arthritis, which mainly affects my ankles (old injury) and thumbs. Repetitive use of my hands can hurt, and my feet will ache after a long day of surgery. In terms of my symptoms, I'm typical of the majority of arthritis sufferers.

So the treatments I'm about to outline are more than just theory or observation. I'm here to tell you that I've actually test-driven all of them myself, and they do work. So come on—let's get started together.

Precaution

One final note before we jump into this chapter—and it's *important*, so listen. Nothing that precedes or follows this statement should be interpreted in any way as replacing a visit to your own doctor, who can take a detailed history and order appropriate tests to determine whether osteoarthritis is in fact cause of your symptoms or you have another disease. (For instance, gout—which, as we've seen, is caused by too much uric acid in the bloodstream—often mimics arthritic symptoms.) So, no excuses—consult your doctor first before embarking on any plan, whether the one described in this book or any other.

Weight Reduction: Seven Strategies That Work

Epidemiological studies have consistently shown the relationship between obesity and osteoarthritis of the knee. Weight reduction has been shown to decrease the risk of arthritis progression as well as improve joint mobility. Weight loss will decrease the impact forces across an arthritic joint on a daily basis. This will lessen inflammation and pain associated with the joint while improving general health.

It is known that patients with early arthritis tend to reduce their physical activity, which causes weight gain, which in turn promotes further wear and tear on the joint. Obesity, especially in women, has been shown to increase knee osteoarthritis, while a weight reduction of about eleven pounds over ten years has been shown to decrease the risk of symptomatic arthritis in women by more than 50 percent. I tell my patients that an extra ten pounds above the waist translates into seventy to one hundred extra pounds of pressure on the knees every time you take a step. And when you consider that on average we take between five thousand and ten thousand steps a day . . . well, you can do the math.

Each year, countless studies investigate various weight loss tactics, such as low-fat diets versus high-fat regimens, whether it's beneficial to snack or not, and the importance of exercise for weight loss and maintenance of a healthy weight. Data from large groups whose members lost weight on their own and kept it off also have been analyzed to determine how those individuals achieved success.

The latest studies conclude that a successful weight loss plan involves not only monitoring calorie intake and expenditure but also dealing with the psychological side of weight loss and habit change. Truly, it's a mind/body undertaking.

But what really works and what doesn't? These seven proven principles can increase your chances of weight loss success now—and for the long term.

1. Get Mentally Prepared Before You Start

Ask yourself two key questions before starting a weight loss program: (1) Compared with the last time you dieted, how motivated are you now? (2) Do you see yourself being committed for the weeks, months, or years it will take to reach your goal?

If you can honestly answer "Very!" to the first question and "Yes!" to the second, you're ready to take on the challenge of weight loss. If you're not mentally prepped before you dive into a diet, you're more likely to mount a halfhearted effort and suffer the inevitable consequence: regaining the weight.

I'm reminded of one particular athlete who was my patient at the USC sports medicine clinic. He had suffered a debilitating basketball injury months before and was now ready to get back in the game. But for the first three games he did everything wrong. His body was ready, but his mind was not—deep down he was afraid of getting injured again. Eventually he was able to face his fear and replace the negative with a positive: continuing his career, winning the admiration of his friends and family as well as his teammates, and, most of all, returning to the game that he truly loved.

If your motivation needs a boost, list the negative aspects of staying at your present weight. These could include increased health risks, low energy, or not looking your best. Then list the positives: better health, more energy, looking better, and the admiration of your friends, family, and colleagues. Keep that list on your refrigerator door and slip a small copy into your wallet. Look at it at least twice daily.

THE PSYCHOLOGY OF
EATING RIGHT (AND WRONG)

A growing body of research is asking why we eat in ways that promote obesity, and we're beginning to find answers in the new field of the psychology of eating.

- **Retrain your brain.** Psychologist Kelly Brownell, director of the Rudd Center for Food Policy and Obesity at Yale University, suggests that at some point over the last couple of decades many Americans lost control of how to eat properly. Former taboos such as eating gargantuan portions, eating throughout the day, and eating late at night have become acceptable. "All the boundaries that would put limits around eating have been exploded," he says. Bottom line: before you start putting food in your mouth, think about how much and when you're eating.

- **Look for support . . . but maybe not at home.** If you're over-weight, chances are your significant other is, too. Studies show that people with higher body mass index (BMI) tend to part-ner with those of similar BMI, and thus may predispose their offspring to obesity. So as much as you may love your beloved co-couch potato, he or she may not be your best partner for losing weight. Seek help and support outside the household.

- **Your iPhone is making you fat.** That may sound ridiculous, but think about it: significant increases in the prevalence of obesity occurred over the past thirty years—just when com-puters and technology use exploded. Being available every waking moment to employers, spouses, children, and others means we're cognitively overloaded. The resulting anxiety just might be wearing down our self-control to resist food temptations. My advice—and this is coming from a surgeon often on call throughout the day—is to incorporate short bursts of time when you turn off the phone, walk away from

(Continues)

THE PSYCHOLOGY OF EATING RIGHT (AND WRONG)
(*Continued*)

the computer, and go off the grid. It might be a five-minute meditation or a quick walk around the block. Clearing your mind will help control your appetite.

- **The buffet effect.** With the advent of the mass production and mass marketing of food came the phenomenon's alter ego—endless variety. Researcher Barbara Rolls has found that something as seemingly innocuous as more variety actually encourages overeating. She says pleasure from eating any particular food declines while you're eating it. But if other foods at the meal have different tastes, aromas, shapes, and textures, instead of stopping eating, people shift to another food that remains appealing. "It's the buffet effect," she says. "If you go to a place with fifty different kinds of foods, you're going to eat more than if there were just a few." Variety might be the spice of life, but it's also an ingredient in obesity. What's a foodie to do? Avoid buffets when eating out, and stick to your grocery list when food shopping.

2. Aim to Lose No More Than 10 Percent of Your Weight in Six Months

Forget trying to be model thin or get down to what you weighed in high school. Set a more modest goal by cutting 3,500 to 7,000 calories per week from what you normally consume. That will give you a weight loss of one to two pounds a week. Even those with life-threatening weight problems are advised to stick to that humble objective. Why?

Research indicates that most people aren't able to lose more than 10 percent of their weight over a six-month period. Even if you could, studies suggest you'd be more likely to gain it back. Losing so little over such a long time may seem like a small thing, but if you keep the weight off, it's a huge achievement.

3. Include Regular Exercise in Your Weight Loss Plan

Studies show that exercise alone doesn't produce much weight loss. To drop pounds, you must reduce your calorie intake as well. Still, you should get in the habit of exercising while in the weight loss phase of your diet because you'll need it when you move to weight maintenance. In study after study, the people who exercise are the people who keep weight off over the long term.

Indeed, in a study of three thousand people who lost at least thirty pounds and kept the weight off for a year or more, 90 percent said exercise was the key to their weight maintenance, according to the National Weight Control Registry. The 2005 dietary guidelines from the US Department of Agriculture recommend thirty to sixty minutes of moderate to vigorous exercise daily to help prevent weight gain, and sixty to ninety minutes daily to help you lose weight. In their book *Younger Next Year*, Chris Crowley and Henry S. Lodge, MD, write that we should exercise six days a week. The exercise work—yes, it's work—will offer significant benefits in the decades ahead. Think of it as your "personal job," akin to your "professional job" in that both require a regular investment of time to see a return—a paycheck in the latter case and good health in the former.

4. Diets and the Law of Thermodynamics

As I write this from my home in Los Angeles, I'm thinking of an article I saw in today's *Los Angeles Times* lifestyle section, which proclaims, "The shelves this summer are full of new weight loss books." A slew of new diet books appear each summer, as regularly as blockbuster films based on comic book characters arrive at the movie theater.

The article reviewed eight diet books released within weeks of each other, each guaranteeing that its brand of eating strategies was the final answer to weight loss. So which is right, the modified paleo diet or the pro-starch one? Is eating gluten-free or skipping breakfast the key to a slimmer you?

Here's what science says: a calorie is still a calorie, whether it comes from fat or carbohydrate or protein. That's the same conclusion reached by the *Lancet* obesity series, whose scientists found that "the body quickly adapts through complex physiological mechanisms underlying metabolic fuel selection."

In other words, changes in diet result in rapid adaptations by the body to match the food selection. These shifts minimize changes in body composition and energy expenditure, and ultimately can torpedo your efforts at weight loss. That's the law of thermodynamics in action in the human body.

Fats supply energy and essential fatty acids, and they help the body absorb the fat-soluble vitamins A, D, E, and K as well as the important nutrients known as carotenoids. Fat contains nine calories per gram; carbohydrates and proteins contain four calories per gram. So one gram of fat gives you more calories than one gram of carbohydrate.

Reducing the amount of fat you eat is one way to limit your overall calorie intake. Eating fat-free or reduced-fat foods isn't always the answer to weight loss, especially if you eat more of the reduced-fat food than you would of the regular item. For example, if you eat twice as many fat-free crackers as regular crackers, you have increased your overall calorie intake. Remember, just because a product is fat-free, it doesn't mean that it is calorie-free. All calories count!

Finally, there's now a consensus among nutritionists on what constitutes a healthful diet that will provide you with the nutrients you need without packing on the weight. It's a whole-food, whole-grain diet that emphasizes lots of fresh fruits and vegetables (of many different colors) and avoids large amounts of animal proteins, sugar, fat, salt, and refined carbohydrates. You can still gain weight on such a diet—again, it's calories in versus calories out. But such an eating plan reduces the amount of high-calorie foods that for most of us represent the slippery slope to overweight and obesity.

5. Avoid Snacking

According to a recent University of North Carolina survey of the eating habits of more than sixty-three thousand people nationwide, Americans' snack consumption has increased more than 50 percent over the last twenty years. Such "snackaholic" habits could be contributing to America's collective weight problem. Snackers eat the same amount at meals as nonsnackers, so they end up eating more total calories, according to a recent study at Cornell University.

6. You Can Eat the Foods You Crave . . . Every Now and Then

On special occasions—let's say that you really want the chocolate cake and ice cream at an office party—go ahead and indulge. A recent survey of 208 people who lost an average of sixty-four pounds and kept it off found that those who are successful at weight loss don't deprive themselves of foods they crave or love. Rather, they have control systems for tempting foods so that they don't go overboard. For example, they'll choose a small slice of cake, along with just a spoonful of ice cream.

7. Weigh Yourself Regularly

Don't ignore your scale and go only by other indicators, such as how well your jeans fit. Instead, play the numbers game and step on the scale once a week.

A weekly weigh-in can accurately help you monitor your weight. If you gain five pounds or more, take immediate action. Ask yourself what you've been doing lately that might have caused the weight gain, then make changes to lose those extra few pounds within the month. Statistics show that people who weigh themselves weekly find it easier to achieve their weight loss goal, because they keep their eye on the ball.

When Food Is an Addiction

For a minority of those who are overweight, food is an addiction. Studies indicate that there is a genetic factor associated with food addiction. Like alcoholics, food addicts just don't know when to stop—their "appetite triggers" are broken. A recent Yale University study found that certain foods, often those containing lots of sugar, salt, or fat, can trigger the same brain receptors that are triggered by addictive drugs. Support programs, particularly twelve-step ones patterned after Alcoholics Anonymous, and cognitive behavioral therapy can help people cope with food addiction.

Exercise: Strategies for Building Muscle and Losing Flab

It used to be that my biggest concern regarding arthritis for those under twenty years of age was sports injuries to joints, which could haunt them later in life. Now it's not that young people exercise too much, but that they don't exercise at all.

The CDC recently reported that one-third of people between the ages of twelve and twenty do not regularly engage in vigorous physical activity. This trend emerged in the 1990s, when budgets for many school physical education programs were slashed. (I also can't help noticing that this is when video games began becoming so popular.)

Not only is exercise key to effective weight control for most people but also it's essential for strengthening your body's muscles—the first line of defense against the symptoms of arthritis. Strong muscles surrounding the joints can alleviate the stress placed on them by deteriorating cartilage. What's more, muscle development improves balance, helping you to avoid falls; the injuries resulting from falls can accelerate the development of debilitating arthritic symptoms.

Alternate Exercise and Rest

If you already have osteoarthritis, exercise must be integrated with periods of rest in the proper balance. Rest will help ease the pain and swelling that you are experiencing. Putting stress on already inflamed joints can accelerate joint damage.

The benefits of exercise for everyone are well established. And while vigorous exercise with an arthritic joint is not often possible, wise and focused exercise is important. Moving all the other joints daily will help keep these joints mobile, giving added support and preventing contractures. Weight-bearing exercises put gentle stress on bones, which increases bone mass, reducing the chances of osteoporosis. This is especially true in the senior set.

Movement of the joint helps nutrients and waste products flow into and out of your articular cartilage, maintaining the health of the joint. Exercise also is a great cardiovascular conditioner, as well as a natural relaxant and mood improver. It will help sleep and aids in the digestion of food. And, as we've seen, a good exercise program will help you control your weight.

Strengthening Muscles

The overall goal of any osteoarthritis exercise program is to maintain motion, preserve strength, and decrease pain. In Chapter 5 I'll describe in much more detail a program of exercise designed to strengthen your muscles and keep your joints functioning in all planes of motion. Here let me emphasize that you should engage in gentle exercise on a daily basis to decrease stiffness and deformity. If you have arthritis, you may not often use your joints through their complete range of motion, and over time the joints can become stiff with contractures; proper exercise that stretches and strengthens muscles will help alleviate this.

If you are doing a regular program of strength training (that is, weight lifting), your muscles will get bigger. It is possible that your overall weight will increase, because muscle weighs more than fat. However, your clothes will probably fit better and your body will be more toned. Your body composition is a better indicator of your overall health than the number on the scale.

If proper technique is followed, most people of any age can safely lift weights. It is important, however, to check with your doctor before you start to train with weights. Also, consult an experienced personal trainer or coach prior to beginning a weight-lifting program. This can help prevent injuries and the loss of muscle strength and endurance that occurs with inactivity.

It is important that people with severe osteoarthritis exercise in a controlled fashion under the supervision of a physical or occupational therapist. Too vigorous a program can actually be harmful to the joint. A qualified therapist can evaluate your entire musculoskeletal system, determining the range of motion of your joints and the strength of your muscles in order to establish a baseline for future physical activity. The therapist can watch your gait and observe how your feet, knees, and hips work together, which will help him or her recommend an appropriate exercise program. Therapists can also recommend aids such as a cane, special shoes, orthotics, or splints. Finally, qualified therapists can help you take into consideration any potential heart problems or other medical issues.

Note that water exercise classes are especially good for arthritic patients, because the buoyancy of water creates less pounding across the joints. If the exercises are done in a heated pool, the heat of the water will also soothe aching muscles. See Chapter 5 for more information on appropriate exercises, including types of water workouts.

Aerobic Exercise

In aerobic exercise, you are continuously moving large muscle groups (such as in your arms, legs, and hips) for a period of time. Your heart rate gets faster and your breathing becomes deeper and faster. All adults should get two and a half hours of aerobic exercise spread out over a week, done in increments of at least ten minutes at a time.

If you have not been active, start slowly and build up over weeks or even months. Walking can be a good exercise to start. Every week, increase the time you spend with the activity, do it more often, or add a second activity. You can increase the speed of your activity or the difficulty of the activity, such as going up hills.

IS RUNNING SAFE?

Intuitively, it might seem that running is bad for arthritis, what with all that pounding on the knee joints. But science does not endorse that hypothesis, and in fact, some studies support the opposite idea: that running not only doesn't contribute to your risk of getting arthritis but also might help you avoid it.

One study conducted at the Stanford University School of Medicine followed a group of long-distance runners for eighteen years. The researchers wanted to know if the runners would experience more severe knee arthritis than their sedentary peers. The results indicated that running did not increase the severity of knee osteoarthritis.

Another study from the University of California at Berkeley involved nearly seventy-five thousand runners over seven years. Those who ran 1.2 miles per day had a 15 percent lower risk of osteoarthritis and a 35 percent lower chance of needing a hip replacement. The researchers concluded that the risk of injuries that might trigger arthritis was reduced by the lower body mass index associated with runners.

That said, if you have an arthritic knee, before beginning a running program you should consult with a medical professional, such as a physical therapist with a sports medicine background who can analyze your gait. Any abnormal joint stress—such as running—can increase the progression of arthritis in an already injured or damaged joint.

Making a Commitment

The decision to keep fit requires a lifelong commitment of time and effort. Exercising and eating right must become things that you do without question, like bathing and brushing your teeth. Unless you are convinced of the benefits, you will not succeed. You're not dabbling in a hobby; what you're really doing is establishing a lifestyle.

Patience is essential. Don't try to do too much too soon, and don't quit before you have a chance to experience the rewards. You can't get back in a few days or weeks what you have lost in years of sedentary living, but you can if you keep at it. And the prize is worth the price.

BONUS HEALTH BENEFITS OF EXERCISE

In addition to strengthening your muscles, regular exercise—even simple walking—decreases your risk of the following:

- Anxiety
- Depression
- Heart attack
- High blood pressure
- Obesity
- Osteoporosis
- Some cancers
- Stroke

Achieving Core Balance Strength

Athletes know this instinctively: strengthening the core muscles is, quite literally, at the center of any optimal exercise program. The midsection and pelvic areas—our "core"—are the body's center of gravity. The core anchors us while we do everything from throwing a baseball to bending down to get the morning paper.

The core consists of three layers of muscles that wrap around our midsection like a natural weight belt. These include the abdominal, hip, lower back, and gluteal muscles. A weak core can contribute to a host of problems, from back pain to bursitis, but also promotes the kind of slip-and-fall accidents that result in fractured hips and broken shoulders, keeping orthopedic surgeons like me busy.

Anyone can do core strength training exercises, because they mimic the body's natural motion and require no special equipment. There are a variety of exercises you can do to strengthen the core, including push-ups, wall squats, V twists, side and circle planks, knee-fold tucks, "climbing rope," sliding pikes, and oblique reaches. These and other exercises can be found online, complete with descriptions, photos, and often videos.

Here's my professional advice: before you begin any core-strengthening regimen, invest in at least two sessions with a qualified, certified personal trainer, physical therapist, or exercise physiologist. This professional can familiarize you with the exercises, and then you can go back and have your coach check your technique again. A qualified expert can also design an exercise regimen specific to your needs and limitations.

The Case for Bariatric Surgery

From the beginning of the book, I told you that I would be completely frank in my advice regarding arthritis. All of my aforementioned advice on losing weight should be tried. But here's the reality: most diets don't work, and once you've reached middle age or a certain weight level, your chances of eating and exercising your way out of obesity diminish further.

Obesity plays such a strong role in arthritis that for patients whose BMI is 35 or above, I can recommend with confidence that bariatric surgery should be considered. (I've mentioned BMI before. It's a universally accepted standard for measuring a person's "fatness," and it takes into account both weight and height. Generally speaking, a BMI of 20 to 25 indicates ideal weight. A BMI over 25 indicates overweight, and a BMI over 30 indicates obesity. Someone with a BMI of 35 or above is classified as clinically or morbidly obese.)

Is bariatric surgery safe? About 220,000 such surgeries are performed annually in the United States. As with any surgical procedure, there's an inherent risk of infection and other complications. Statistically, however, the surgical complication rate for adjustable gastric banding surgery, the most popular bariatric procedure, is fairly low—about the same as for having a gallbladder removed.

The medical establishment, once aghast at the thought of weight loss surgery except in the most extreme cases, has finally seen the light.

In February 2011, the US Food and Drug Administration (FDA) gave the nod to expand eligibility requirements for gastric banding surgery to those with a BMI of 35 (or 30, if they have associated problems such as high blood pressure or diabetes), making twenty-seven million more Americans candidates for this surgery.

If you're morbidly obese and for years have tried dieting and exercising but have had no success, then consider bariatric surgery. The alternative is a continued lifetime of obesity and the prospect of accelerated declining health, including arthritis.

Think of it this way: if you're clinically obese, you're carrying around approximately seventy-five to a hundred or more pounds of excess weight, all of which is grinding down the cartilage between your joints, in particular in your knees. You've heard the phrase "carrying around an extra spare tire" to describe a person's chubbiness? In this case, being morbidly obese is like quite literally carrying around two tires from an average full-size automobile.

Fortunately, bariatric surgery has advanced dramatically over the last five years. Almost a million gastric banding surgeries have been performed laparoscopically since the device was introduced ten years ago, and the procedures have only gotten better—safer and more effective—with time. Essentially, the surgical procedure involves cinching the upper part of the stomach with a plastic band that has a buckle. Through a minute port that extends into the patient's abdomen, the band can be adjusted. This squeezing of the stomach creates a sense of fullness and reduces appetite.

If you're both diabetic (especially severely diabetic) *and* clinically obese, consider an alternative procedure: gastric bypass. The surgery is more involved and potentially more dangerous than gastric banding, but it's the only known bariatric surgery that can treat the symptoms of type 2 diabetes. In fact, it's the only known cure.

Diabetes is an insidious, progressive disease in which the patient's health declines over time. Insulin and other medications slow the decline, but no diabetic patient was ever cured with medications. And medications for diabetes, while they stabilize blood sugar, often result in other ailments, such as kidney failure.

The beauty of gastric bypass surgery is that in most cases there's a complete remission of diabetes symptoms and the patient experiences dramatic weight loss. The mystery is how exactly it works to control diabetes. The best research indicates that a hormonal mechanism becomes defective in diabetic patients, preventing them from processing insulin in the body properly. Gastric bypass surgery literally bypasses the defective hormonal mechanism that appears to be at the root of the problem.

I'm throwing up a cautionary yellow flag here, so take note. The field of bariatric surgery has been invaded lately by marketing companies promoting gastric banding surgery through mass media—as if they were selling the latest soft drink. I'm speaking of TV commercials, online banner ads, and even billboards, all with grinning models who probably never had an ounce of extra weight on their beautiful bodies in the first place. What's more, the physicians associated with such marketing are often not qualified to perform bariatric surgery. A degree in medicine is not an all-access backstage pass for all types of surgery. I have been a practicing surgeon for thirty years, but my specialty is orthopedics—I'm not qualified to perform bariatric surgery.

HOW TO CHOOSE A
QUALIFIED BARIATRIC SURGEON

Weight loss surgery is reserved for the seriously overweight who have tried other methods of weight loss and failed. If you decide to proceed with bariatric surgery, understand that healthy living habits are the key to success. Weight loss surgery is the proverbial quick fix, but by no means is it a permanent solution by itself. Accept that you'll have to change the way you eat and the way you live after bariatric surgery, and keep it up for the rest of your life.

(Continues)

**HOW TO CHOOSE A QUALIFIED
BARIATRIC SURGEON** (*Continued*)

Here are some questions to consider before embarking upon weight loss surgery:

- *Which procedure is best for you?* If you and your physician determine that weight loss surgery is appropriate then you must next decide which surgical procedure is your best option. By all means, empower yourself by doing your own research and talk to people who have already had weight loss surgery. Ultimately, however, you will need to consult an expert bariatric surgeon.

- *How do you choose a surgeon who's qualified?* At a bare minimum, your surgeon should be certified by the American Society for Metabolic and Bariatric Surgery and the American Board of Surgery. Your surgeon should be able to provide you with the number of operations he or she has performed and the complication rates. Choose a surgeon who has participated in research related to weight loss surgery. Ideally, you want a surgeon who is capable of doing more than just gastric banding operations, someone who has the expertise to perform a wide variety of complex laparoscopic abdominal operations.

- *The multidisciplinary approach.* Along with choosing a qualified surgeon, it is imperative to select a program that offers a multidisciplinary group of health professionals including physicians, nurses, dietitians, and mental health specialists. Obesity is a complex disease that requires a comprehensive support program, from initial consultations to surgery to extensive aftercare.

- *What services does the program provide to ensure your success?* Surgery is a tool. As I've said, by itself it is not adequate for long-term success. Keeping weight off over the long term after surgery requires a comprehensive, fully integrated treatment plan. Look for a program that offers classes in nutrition, support groups, help in establishing a fitness regimen, educational talks, and other therapeutic programs. It's an approach that encompasses all aspects of health and wellness for the long term . . . a program for life.

Takeaways

In this chapter, we've seen that weight management and exercise are vital in avoiding obesity and the early onset of arthritis symptoms. Strengthening muscles around the joints can help alleviate the natural loss of cartilage that comes with age, while shedding excess pounds reduces the pressure around the joints. Aerobic exercise can promote weight loss.

The key to both exercise and weight management is the law of thermodynamics as it applies to the human body: for weight to be stable, the number of calories we consume should be equal to the number of calories we burn. Maintaining the right energy balance is easier if you eat a healthful diet rich in whole grains and fresh fruits and vegetables and avoid sugar, fats, simple carbs, and salt (the formula for junk food).

One last piece of advice about the importance of a well-formulated diet and exercise regimen in treating arthritis: don't expect your doctor to recommend one. A recent report found that many doctors in the United States simply don't think to recommend exercise and weight loss to help treat their patients' osteoarthritis, instead focusing on pain-relieving drugs and surgery.

If you're already obese, especially morbidly obese, and if realistically you're not likely to exercise in a meaningful way, consult with your physician about considering weight loss surgery as an option. Weight loss is a long-term lifestyle choice.

4

THE WILD WEST OF
ARTHRITIS SUPPLEMENTS

Google "arthritis supplements" and you get tens of thousands of results. It's a tidal wave of claims and counterclaims, largely unregulated by the government. But don't stop with the virtual world. Supplements are available in a wide variety of retail outlets, from the GNC store at the local mall to the neighborhood Trader Joe's.

Exactly how did we get to this Wild West of osteoarthritis medications? Most of it is a result of the seemingly haphazard way the federal government regulates drugs in general, classifying some as "prescription" (available only through a licensed physician) and others as "over-the-counter" (available to anyone). It's a distinction that in many cases cannot really determine a particular drug's effectiveness or safety. To be clear, while you may think some government or scientific entity must be overseeing what goes into the myriad of over-the-counter (OTC) supplements, the reality is that the sheriff is permanently out to lunch.

Does that mean all natural supplements are bad? Not necessarily. In fact, some say there is research to back up their claims. But caveat emptor. Often these studies are administered, financed, and reviewed by the supplement manufacturer, with no objective third-party involvement.

Even the most studied of the supplements, glucosamine and chondroitin, have produced inconclusive findings. Random clinical trials are the basis for evidence-based medicine, but OTC supplements are sorely lacking in these kinds of scientific studies.

Practically the only time the FDA, the government's main regulatory agency for all things concerning drugs and food, gets involved with natural supplements is when a product is suspected of being tainted. That is, when someone gets sick or dies from one of them, the FDA issues a warning or directive. Needless to say, that might be a tad too late if you were the unlucky customer who got the bad supplement.

Beyond product safety concerns, you should always be cautious about self-medicating, even with something as benign-sounding as "natural supplements." If you take too much of a seemingly good thing, you could easily wind up with toxic levels of the ingredient in your system. Also, some OTC supplements react adversely with prescription medications or with each other. Bottom line: speak with your health care professional (doctor or pharmacist) before embarking on a regimen of OTC supplements.

Glucosamine and Chondroitin

Two of the most promising supplements, and certainly the most studied of the lot, are glucosamine and chondroitin. They are marketed and sold as standalone products, in combination with each other, and in combination with other ingredients.

Integral elements of the cartilaginous matrix, glucosamine and chondroitin were recognized for their medicinal value as far back as 1969. These compounds have been used liberally in Europe and Asia during the past fifteen years to treat arthritis. Public interest in the United States gained momentum after the 1997 publication of the book *The Arthritis Cure*, by Jason Theodosakis, Brenda Adderly, and Barry Fox, which described the disease-modifying properties of these substances and their ability to offer symptomatic relief with few side effects.

Despite the curiosity aroused by these supplements, little is known about how they work in the body, and their role in the treatment of osteoarthritis has not been scientifically substantiated. The Arthritis Foundation maintains a neutral position regarding their use, stating that because scientific evidence is lacking, they cannot be recommended as a first-line treatment. The American Academy of Orthopaedic Surgeons does not think they are a proven treatment. Marketed as nutritional supplements, they do not have to undergo the same rigorous testing as pharmaceuticals. Critics caution that their long-term efficacy and safety are unknown, and advise that until better information is available, they should be used in moderation. To date, there have been no data suggesting they are harmful.

Although there is some evidence that glucosamine and chondroitin can influence cartilage metabolism, most information comes from in vitro models or animal studies. The effects seen in such studies have not been established in human studies yet, nor has it been shown that the metabolic responses found in these preliminary studies occur in older or arthritic cartilage as well. Thus we have to take with a grain of salt proponents' claims that glucosamine and chondroitin are cartilage-protecting agents with matrix-modifying properties.

Both agents seem to have more than one mechanism of action. There is some indication that they may stimulate the production of the elements of cartilage and down-regulate the production of proteolytic enzymes that can destroy cartilage. These products have also been associated with improved synovial fluid characteristics and anti-inflammatory properties. Although it is unclear if these effects are physiologically relevant, they warrant additional investigation.

Glucosamine Alone

Several placebo-controlled trials in the early 1980s performed by European and Asian researchers appear to show that glucosamine reduces pain and improves range of motion. In one study comparing glucosamine supplements to a placebo, 73.3 percent of patients taking the glucosamine improved throughout the thirty-day study, versus 41.3 percent of those who took the placebo. Other placebo-controlled trials, using oral, intramuscular, and even intra-articular glucosamine products, demonstrated that glucosamine produces better and longer-lasting pain relief, improved range of motion, and (to a lesser extent) greater reduction of swelling than a placebo.

Comparison studies with glucosamine and nonsteroidal anti-inflammatory drugs have shown favorable results, with glucosamine offering a delayed but progressive and longer-lasting effect. One study compared glucosamine sulfate to ibuprofen using the Lequesne index, which assesses pain, walking, and activities of daily living. Although all patients showed good to moderate results based on these criteria, there was no significant difference between the two groups at the end of the study. Consistent with the results of the comparison study mentioned at the beginning of this paragraph, the patients in the ibuprofen group did respond more rapidly, with 48 percent showing a response within one week, versus 28 percent of patients in the glucosamine group. An important factor to consider is the adverse effects associated with ibuprofen, such as gastrointestinal, kidney, and liver disorders.

Glucosamine hydrochloride was also tested during an eight-week study of 118 patients with knee osteoarthritis. A daily diary maintained by each patient revealed significantly less pain with glucosamine than with placebo, and range of motion was significantly better at the end of the study with glucosamine.

Finally, in an attempt to demonstrate glucosamine's ability to protect cartilage from degradation, several studies that have X-rayed patients with arthritic knees have shown that patients taking glucosamine experience far less joint space narrowing than the placebo group. That is, glucosamine appeared to reduce the progression of cartilage deterioration.

Chondroitin Alone

Although chondroitin sulfate typically is marketed as a co-ingredient with glucosamine, there are products that contain chondroitin as the sole ingredient and claim to have beneficial effects on the symptoms of osteoarthritis. Several trials were done in the 1990s to determine the benefits of chondroitin sulfate, and their conclusions, consistent with the glucosamine studies, are that chondroitin is effective against osteo-arthritis in reducing pain and improving joint function.

A more recent study demonstrated chondroitin's ability to signifi-cantly reduce the number of joints that show osteoarthritic erosions, despite the inability to halt the progression of the disease in a specific joint. Though studies on rabbits have demonstrated a reduction in joint space narrowing similar to that seen with glucosamine, more studies are needed to evaluate the structure-modifying capabilities of chondroitin.

Combination of Glucosamine and Chondroitin

Experimental studies have demonstrated a synergistic effect when glu-cosamine and chondroitin are administered together. Because each of these agents has a different mechanism of action, the body appears to respond best when the two are taken simultaneously.

One scientific study of military personnel evaluated the effectiveness of Cosamine, a product combining glucosamine, chondroitin, manga-nese, and vitamin C, in treating patients with knee osteoarthritis and patients with degeneration of the spine. Significant improvements were seen only in the patients with knee pain.

In 2005 the National Institutes of Health conducted the Glucos-amine/Chondroitin Arthritis Intervention Trial (GAIT), a large, mul-timillion-dollar, randomized, placebo-controlled study, at several sites across the United States—the largest test of these supplements carried out to date. It involved the following groups: placebo, chondroitin with glucosamine, glucosamine alone, chondroitin alone, and NSAIDs.

The results? In a word, disappointing. Overall, there were no sig-nificant differences between the treatments tested and placebo. For a subset of participants with moderate to severe pain, glucosamine com-bined with chondroitin sulfate provided statistically significant pain relief compared with placebo—about 79 percent of those taking the combination had a 20 percent or greater reduction in pain versus about 54 percent for placebo. The study's data were reevaluated in 2010, with the same results: patients with moderate to severe pain seemed to have benefited measurably, if not to a hugely significant degree.

The current scientific literature on the effectiveness of these products has been criticized for numerous reasons. These products have not been subjected to the rigorous testing protocols of the FDA or other agencies because they are considered not medicines but rather dietary supplements. Because dietary supplements cannot be patented, according to the Dietary Supplement Health and Education Act of 1984, pharmaceutical companies have not been inclined to assist in testing of glucosamine and chondroitin. Most funding for the published outcome studies has therefore come from the product manufacturers and commercial sponsorship. The Arthritis Foundation acknowledges glucosamine and chondroitin's ability to both relieve pain and slow cartilage damage, but it recognizes that these results have been substantiated only in some people. It currently recommends the accepted daily doses of 1,500 mg for glucosamine and 1,200 mg for chondroitin. It doesn't matter which form of either supplement you take; all produce essentially the same results. The Arthritis Foundation suggests that patients discontinue the products if symptoms do not improve within a few months. However, those people who say that a combination of glucosamine and chondroitin works for them also note that it appears to take many weeks to work.

Safety

It appears that glucosamine and chondroitin are safe to use, with minor adverse effects such as gastrointestinal complaints, headache, leg pain and swelling, and itching being reported. It is not known whether long-term use would have any physiologic consequences.

There is evidence that glucosamine affects the metabolism of glucose and insulin. It is not completely understood how this occurs, nor is it known what dose of glucosamine is needed to have this effect. Another experiment found that infusion of glucosamine in normal rats resulted in resistance to insulin stimulation of glucose uptake and glycogen synthesis in skeletal muscle. Other studies have raised concerns regarding glucosamine and its effect on varying mechanisms of insulin resistance. While there's been no correlation of these findings to people, still they should give pause to patients with diabetes.

Since the Dietary Supplement Health and Education Act does not require the same manufacturing and processing guidelines for nutritional supplements as for pharmaceuticals, many supplements may not contain high-quality ingredients or even the labeled quantity of ingredients. In fact, studies of commercial glucosamine products have shown that the supplements contain from 59 percent to 138 percent of the dosage stated on the product label. Patients and physicians should choose brands with proven effectiveness and high quality standards.

Recommendation

The primary criticism seen in the literature on glucosamine and chondroitin involves length of follow-up and the lack of long-term outcome data. Additionally, although specific doses of specific forms of glucosamine and chondroitin have been tested, the market supplies products with varying purity, compound structure, and combinations that have not been specifically investigated. Although side effects have been few and relatively benign, the consequences of extended use of chondroitin and glucosamine are not known. They appear to have pain-relieving properties and they're relatively inexpensive, but to date their efficacy has not been irrefutably substantiated.

We do not yet know definitely in which patients these products might work, what the indications are for their use, and which patients may be at risk because of their use. As Stephen Owens, Phillip Wagner, and I wrote in an article for the *Journal of Knee Surgery*, "The American medical community desires a more critical evaluation of these agents through better controlled and better engineered studies."

Based on my own clinical experience with the two supplements, it appears they do help many patients with pain management. That, along with significant if not definitive evidence that they do no harm and might help slow the degradation of cartilage, leads me to make this recommendation: try a combination of the two for three months and see if you notice a difference in pain and mobility.

Herbs, Spices, and Plants

If the case for using glucosamine and chondroitin seems less than convincing, better buckle your seat belt for the bumpy road ahead. All other supplements that promise to help arthritis sufferers pale in comparison in terms of the science behind them. In other words, there's very little to no credible research to back their claims.

The one that comes closest to having been supported by at least some science is S-adenosylmethionine (SAM-e), a compound produced naturally in the body. Your liver makes it from the amino acid methionine, and it plays an essential role in the formation of hormones, neurotransmitters, and phospholipids.

Some manufacturers' studies indicate that SAM-e may help encourage the production of cartilage cells and increase cartilage thickness. SAM-e has been found to be effective as anti-inflammatory painkillers in treating osteoarthritis, but with fewer side effects. A recent trial comparing SAM-e with the drug Celebrex showed no difference between the two in terms of pain relief after two months of treatment (although it may be necessary to take SAM-e for up to thirty days before noticeable relief occurs).

Although SAM-e is considered safe, it may not be for people taking medication for bipolar or depressive disorder. These individuals must watch for drug interactions, since SAM-e can affect serotonin levels. Do not take it with dextromethorphan (a cough suppressant found in Robitussin DM and other products), medications for depression, medications for Parkinson's disease, Demerol (meperidine), Talwin (pentazocine), or Ultram (tramadol).

Here are the ABCs of the other leading over-the-counter supplements promoted for osteoarthritis treatment. Again, there is very little evidence proving the effectiveness of any of these.

ASU is the acronym sometimes used for **unsaponifiable avocado soybean** (see below).

Autumn crocus is a plant whose seed, bulb, and flower are used in folk medicine. Despite serious safety concerns, autumn crocus is used for gouty arthritis and an inherited disease called familial Mediterranean fever. The seeds of autumn crocus contain colchicine, which purport-edly reduces the chemicals that cause joint swelling in people with these diseases. Although colchicine is considered highly effective for treating acute gouty arthritis, it is not effective for all types of pain. Colchicine is not considered an analgesic (painkilling) drug.

Bromelain, found in pineapple, is an enzyme with anti-inflamma-tory properties that may or may not be effective for the treatment of osteoarthritis. However, when combined with rutin (see below) and trypsin (a pancreatic enzyme), it may help in reducing osteoarthritis pain and improving knee function. Bromelain is safe for most people, but side effects have been reported, including stomach discomfort. It may also cause an allergic reaction, particularly in people who have other allergies. It is available in capsules or tablets.

Camphor comes from the wood of a species of large Asian ever-green tree. A topical cream containing camphor, glucosamine sulfate, and chondroitin sulfate seems to reduce the severity of arthritic pain by about half; researchers believe that the counterirritant effects of the camphor, not the other ingredients, cause this relief.

Cat's claw is a tropical vine that grows in rain forest and jungle areas. It is taken to relieve knee pain related to physical activity. How-ever, it does not reduce knee swelling or decrease pain when resting. Studies indicate that cat's claw has no significant side effects.

Devil's claw is a plant native to southern Africa. Taking it either alone or with anti-inflammatory drugs seems to help in decreasing osteoarthritis pain. The most common side effect is diarrhea (experi-enced by about 8 percent of people participating in one research study). Other possible side effects include nausea, vomiting, abdominal pain, headaches, ringing in the ears, loss of appetite, and loss of taste. It can also cause allergic skin reactions, menstrual problems, and changes in blood pressure.

DMSO (dimethyl sulfoxide) is a clear liquid that is externally applied, injected, or ingested orally. However, it has some rather unpleasant side effects. The most notable is that it leaves a very bad taste in the mouth, and the breath will have a pronounced odor of garlic and oysters. When it was first introduced in the 1960s, studies on animals indicated that it was causing damage to the lens of the eye. There is no evidence that the same holds true for humans, but these findings quickly caused DMSO to fall from favor. It resurfaced with the running boom in the 1970s and 1980s as a topical treatment for sore muscles. The most eye-opening aspect of DMSO is that it can be found at most hardware stores, because it's also used as a solvent; clearly, only a purified form should be used in humans. Because of these reasons, DMSO is rarely used for treating osteoarthritis today.

Feverfew is a perennial herb that has been used for centuries to treat ailments such as headache and joint pain. The botanical name for feverfew is *Tanacetum parthenium,* but the plant is known by several common names, such as featherfew, midsummer daisy, and wild chamomile. Feverfew grows in Europe as well as North and South America and has been used for centuries in folk medicine as well as traditional medicine to relieve pain and treat various ailments. However, more research is needed to determine the effectiveness of feverfew in treating osteoarthritis. Although laboratory tests demonstrate the anti-inflammatory properties of feverfew, it was no more effective than a placebo in a study of individuals with rheumatoid arthritis. Feverfew supplements are available in capsule, tablet, and liquid forms. Feverfew may interact with blood-thinning medications and can increase the tendency to bleed.

Fish oil, which comes in a variety of different products and forms, is believed by proponents to fight cytokines that destroy joint tissue, but there is no scientific evidence to support these claims.

Flaxseed oil is derived from the seed of the *Linum usitatissimum* plant and used to decrease the inflammation and pain of osteoarthritis. It is safe for most adults but may cause slow blood clotting or lower blood pressure. Flaxseed oil is used for many conditions, but so far there isn't enough scientific evidence to determine whether it is effective for any of them.

Ginger originates from the root of the ginger plant. It contains active ingredients that may have analgesic (pain-relieving) and anti-inflammatory properties. Warnings are associated with ginger; notably, it can interfere with medications for blood thinning.

Green tea is made from unfermented leaves of *Camellia sinensis* and has been consumed for years for its powerful antioxidant properties and medicinal value. In addition to osteoarthritis, green tea is purportedly helpful for joint inflammation, cancer, weight loss, liver problems, diabetes, and inflammatory bowel disease. For osteoarthritis inflammation, the University of Maryland Medical Center suggests preparing green tea by mixing one to two teaspoons of leaves into a cup of boiling water and letting it steep for at least ten minutes.

Instaflex is a commercial product that its maker designed to be an all-encompassing joint solution, bringing together several supplements in one product. The product launched in the summer of 2010 in the United States exclusively in GNC stores. There are four formulations of Instaflex: Joint Support, Bone Support, Muscle Support, and Multivitamin. Instaflex Joint Support contains eight active ingredients: 1,500 mg glucosamine sulfate, 500 mg methylsulfonylmethane (MSM), 250 mg white willow bark extract (standardized to 15 percent salicin), 250 mg gingerroot concentrate 4:1, 125 mg *Boswellia serrata* extract (standardized to 65 percent boswellic acid), 50 mg turmeric root extract (standardized to 95 percent curcumin), 50 mg cayenne 40mhu, and 4 mg hyaluronic acid. No scientific studies support that this combination of ingredients in those amounts is effective in treating arthritic symptoms.

MSM (methylsulfonylmethane) is a naturally occurring compound found in small amounts in fresh foods, including fruits, vegetables, legumes, milk, eggs, fish, and grains. When foods are processed or heated, however, MSM is destroyed. In supplement form, MSM is usually derived from sulfur-rich plant or tree fibers. Some preliminary research suggests that MSM can modestly reduce some symptoms of osteoarthritis such as pain and swelling. MSM has not been shown to significantly reduce stiffness. It is considered safe and well tolerated with side effects comparable to those of placebo; however, clinical trials have not been long-term.

Pycnogenol is an antioxidant extracted from the bark of the French maritime pine tree. It has been found to contain procyanidins, bioflavonoids, and organic acids, all of which reportedly enhance good health naturally. Pycnogenol has been studied for the past thirty-five years and has been found to be safe. It contains natural compounds called procyanidolic oligomers that are supposed to help maintain integrity of the joints by fighting free radicals. The antioxidant activity of procyanidolic oligomers is fifty times greater than the antioxidant activity of vitamin C or vitamin E. Pycnogenol is available in more than six hundred dietary supplements, vitamins, and other health products.

Resveratrol is a natural compound with anti-inflammatory properties that is usually considered as a therapy for rheumatoid arthritis. Known to have antimicrobial properties as well as to offer cardiovascular protection, resveratrol is found in high levels in the skins of grapes and also in red wine. At least two studies indicate that it may interrupt the inflammatory cascade that degrades cartilage in osteoarthritis.

Rose hips are the seedpods of roses. Rose hips have become a popular natural treatment for arthritis. They contain anthocyanins, plant compounds found to have antioxidant properties. As a supplement, rose hips have been used for relief of OA pain; however, they have not been approved for treating any joint condition. Rose hips are available as an oil as well as in powder or capsule form.

Rutin is found in buckwheat, citrus fruits, black tea, and apple peels. When taken in combination with bromelain and trypsin, it appears to reduce pain and improve knee function in some arthritis sufferers. Rutin supplements can be found in capsule or pill form or can be injected into the body as a liquid. Despite the various uses of rutin, it is important to be aware of side effects associated with it. These can include a high white blood cell count, skin rashes, hair loss, vomiting, constipation, diarrhea, abdominal pain, dry mouth, sleeping problems, headaches, dizziness, fatigue, muscle stiffness, swelling, and flulike symptoms.

Stinging nettle is a flowering stalklike plant that is found in the United States, Canada, Asia, and Europe. It gets its name from the hairs found on the plant. When touched, the hairs break off and inject themselves into the skin, releasing a combination of chemicals that produces a painful stinging sensation. The leaves have been used in folk medicine precisely because of that effect—placed on a painful area of the body, they can relieve the pain in that area. It is believed that the chemicals released by the hairs of the stinging nettle interrupt the pain receptors and possibly decrease the inflammatory chemicals in the painful area. Its medicinal history goes back to medieval Europe, when it was used as a diuretic and to relieve joint pain in osteoarthritis patients. Stinging nettle can be taken internally as well as used topically and also is available in tea form, as whole leaves, as a tincture, as an extract, and in capsules.

Tart cherry juice was found to significantly reduce inflammatory markers, according to study results presented at the 2012 American College of Sports Medicine conference. The study, conducted by researchers from Oregon Health and Science University, involved twenty women between the ages of forty and seventy who had osteoarthritis. Anthocyanins are the compounds that give tart cherries their vibrant color, high antioxidant level, and ability to reduce inflammation. Previous studies have linked the fruit to decreased joint and muscle pain. In this study, researchers found that up to 40 percent of osteoarthritis patients have inflammation, and "tart cherries may provide beneficial anti-inflammatory activity helping osteoarthritis patients manage their disease." Tart cherry juice reportedly was seen being taken by lots of athletes at the London Olympics in 2012.

Thunder god vine is an ancient herb that has been used in traditional Chinese medicine for autoimmune conditions such as rheumatoid arthritis. It's not applicable for osteoarthritis.

Turmeric is an ancient herb used in traditional Indian medicinal systems, not to mention cooking. Like thunder god vine, it is used mainly for rheumatoid arthritis.

Unsaponifiable avocado soybean (also referred to as ASU) is a natural vegetable extract made from avocado and soybean oils. As a dietary supplement, ASU has shown some promise in clinical studies, appearing to significantly reduce the pain associated with osteoarthritis and stimulate cartilage repair. Studies indicate it is most effective for patients suffering from hip pain. A two-year clinical trial on hip osteoarthritis revealed that 300 mg once a day of ASU did not slow down joint space narrowing, and no other significant differences were observed when compared with placebo after one year. A later analysis of the study, however, determined that ASU might decrease joint space narrowing in patients with very severe hip osteoarthritis. ASU took at least two months before any improvement was noticed, according to the study results. Residual symptom relief can be expected for two months after stopping treatment.

Vitamin D has been studied, and results indicated that elderly men with low levels of vitamin D have an increased risk of developing hip osteoarthritis. Other studies offered conflicting results regarding vitamin D and knee osteoarthritis. Some found that low vitamin D levels may cause greater knee pain and difficulty walking in patients with osteoarthritis of the knee. While it's all being sorted out, find out what your vitamin D level is and discuss this supplement with your doctor.

Vitamin E supplementation may be helpful for the symptoms of osteoarthritis; however, the evidence for this is far from conclusive. Much more research needs to be done before it can be recommended as a viable treatment for OA symptoms. Foods that contain the largest amounts of vitamin E include sunflower seeds, almonds, peanut butter, spinach, collard greens, tomatoes, mangos, avocados, broccoli, and blueberries.

Yucca is a plant found in southwestern deserts of the United States and Mexico. The root is eaten as a vegetable and used for medicinal purposes. It is rich in steroidlike saponins that elevate the body's production of cortisone, which can address the pain of certain inflammatory conditions such as osteoarthritis and rheumatoid arthritis. It has been speculated that the saponins block the release of toxins in the intestines that inhibit normal formation of cartilage. However, yucca's ability to relieve symptoms of osteoarthritis has not been widely studied.

Takeaways

Because OTC supplements are not regulated by the government in the same way as pharmaceutical drugs are, they're held to much lower standards in terms of having to prove their effectiveness and safety. True, many of these herbs and spices have been used for millennia in folk medicine. But questions remain about whether they work at all, how effective they may be if they do work, and how they might work. In my own clinical experience, I have seen many patients have good results with the most scientifically studied of the lot, glucosamine and chondroitin. In general these supplements are randomized clinical human trials to validate efficacy.

5

ARTHRITIS EXERCISE
AND DIET STRATEGIES

In Chapter 3 we briefly discussed diet and exercise for weight management. In this chapter, we'll dig deeper into exercise strategies for living with osteoarthritis. The chapter concludes with a discussion of the potential benefits of an anti-inflammatory diet and exactly what science has to say about it.

Here's the truth about exercise and diet: if you were to focus only on diet and embrace a sedentary lifestyle, you still could manage your weight effectively. For the average person, thirty minutes of brisk walking burns just 100 calories—less than half of the calories in a regular two-ounce Snickers candy bar, which has 270 calories. You don't need exercise for weight management. Sure, an active exercise regimen makes it easier to lose weight by speeding up your metabolism. But the inarguable fact is that you don't have to exercise in order to lose weight and maintain that weight loss.

A recent anthropological study from Hunter College looked at the Hadza, a group of indigenous hunter-gatherers in northern Tanzania. In their traditional lifestyle, the Hadza track prey for miles every day, so obviously they engage in a much more physically active lifestyle than the average Western white-collar worker. Yet when at rest, the Hadza burn fewer calories than an office-cubicle dweller. This may be a case in which evolutionary genetics has stepped in and prevented the Hadza from becoming too slender by lowering their calorie-burning thermo-stat while at rest. So when it comes to burning calories through motion, it's pretty much a wash between hunter-gatherers and Internet surfers. Why, then, are we hefty and the Hadza svelte? For one thing, they eat much less than Westerners. And their diet, consisting mainly of lean meat and fresh fruit, contains none of the processed grains, sugar, and fat that permeate our high-calorie junk food.

If our goal is only to lose weight, the message from Chapter 3 remains the same: consume fewer calories. Our goal, however, is more than achieving optimal weight. We want to be fit as well, and this is where regular exercise should become a high priority for anyone living with osteoarthritis. We want not only to prevent the worsening of osteoarthritic symptoms but actually to improve the quality of life.

Now, before we go on with this discussion, let's qualify it. If your arthritis is debilitating at the moment—if it's limiting your range of motion and you find it hard to walk, climb stairs, or even get out of bed—then I want you to first consult with your doctor or phys-ical therapist before trying any of the recommended exercises. You can make an arthritic condition worse by not performing an exercise properly, and in some cases you should not perform a particular exer-cise at all.

You may also have one or more chronic diseases besides arthritis. A 2012 CDC report found that more than one in five Americans between the ages of forty-five and sixty-four have more than one chronic dis-ease, while Americans over sixty-five have a 45 percent chance of having more than one chronic disease. More than half of those who suffer from diabetes, for example, also suffer from arthritis. (Indeed, new research suggests that diabetes independently predicts severe osteoarthritis.) So it's especially important to consult with a medical professional if you suffer from arthritis and another chronic condition before embarking on a new exercise or diet regimen.

But everyone—no matter how severe the arthritis—does need to keep his or her body in motion every day, even if it's just walking around the block. That's a given in any successful arthritis treatment.

So let's jump into our exercise program with the understanding that not every exercise described below might be right for you.

Exercise

Science is clear about this: regular physical activity provides important short-term health benefits and reduces the long-term risk of disability and premature death. Regular physical activity substantially reduces the risk of dying of coronary heart disease, the nation's leading cause of death. Exercise will also decrease the risk of colon cancer, diabetes, and high blood pressure.

Regular activity can help control weight and contribute to the maintenance of healthy bones, muscles, and joints. Exercise can reduce the symptoms of anxiety and depression. For people with arthritis, physical activity has been proven to help relieve pain and maintain joint mobility. There's even evidence that exercise can change how our DNA is expressed: a single twenty-minute workout can induce alterations in gene expression that help muscles work better.

Even with these proven benefits, more than 60 percent of American adults do not engage in the level of physical activity necessary to provide health benefits. More than 25 percent are not active at all in their leisure time, and on average, leisure-time activity decreases with age.

A Fitness Lifestyle

I have a theory about why Americans are so sedentary. Most of us think exercise has to be strenuous and uncomfortable to be effective. I call it the "Manteo Mitchell fear factor." Who's Manteo Mitchell? During the London Olympics in 2012, he was the American runner who helped his team win the gold in the four-hundred-meter relay by finishing the race with a broken leg. The idea is that to be good at exercise you have to be willing to grin and bear extreme pain—even a broken leg. Right?

Well, here's the truth about that old exercise mantra "no pain, no gain": it's true—*if* you're a competitive athlete, and especially if you're an elite athlete striving for a world record. Manteo Mitchell's performance was heroic by any standard, but in fact it wasn't the first of its kind. In 2009 a high school sprinter in New Orleans, Matt Schwingshakl, managed to complete the final eighty meters of his four-hundred-meter race with a broken leg, too. While breaking any bone in the leg is painful, the bones in question in these two cases were not weight-bearing, so the racers indeed could finish their races.

So how did they overcome the pain? They were used to it. When you're a competitive athlete you live with pain all the time. When you're pushing your body to extreme physical activity in the quest to shave one-tenth of a second off your time so that you can be the next Olympic gold medalist, you live with pain. It's part of the job description. You wake up with pain and go to sleep with it. In other words, you deal with it. This is especially true of sports such as football, track and field, and basketball, where the constant strain on weight-bearing joints exponentially increases the chance for major injury.

From my direct observation of athletes for two decades now, the main difference between the also-ran and the champion athlete is how much pain each can—and is willing to—endure. Once you reach a certain level of competition, differences in body type and natural athletic ability are negligible. Who wins and who doesn't has as much to do with mental toughness as it does with physical prowess, and that includes the ability to endure pain.

Malcolm Gladwell, the best-selling author of *Outliers: The Story of Success* and other science-oriented nonfiction works, recently recounted how in his youth he was an elite athlete. No kidding! Born of a white British mother and black Jamaican father, Gladwell was raised in Canada. In the 1970s there were lots of Jamaicans who immigrated to Canada, and Canadian track-and-field events were dominated by young Jamaican émigrés. When Gladwell was thirteen he was so good that he was considered the fastest Canadian of his age group. So why didn't we ever see Gladwell compete in the Olympic Games? At the age of fourteen he threw in the towel. He explained that he was tired of all the pain associated with competitive athletics even at the high school level. He loved running, but he loved other things as well, including writing, and he was not willing to endure the pain of racing and training to stick with it. (As a huge fan of his writing, I'd say we all lucked out with his boyhood decision.)

Athletes at the University of Southern California compete on a world stage: 23 percent of all the US medalists at the 2012 London Olympics were from USC, grabbing 24 of the 104 gold, silver, and bronze medals. But while these elite athletes have to live with pain (though those of us in the sports medicine program certainly try to alleviate it), you and I *don't* have to deal with pain to be physically active. So banish forever those thoughts of Manteo Mitchell, and simply think about what it takes to keep your body fit.

One thing we can borrow from athletes about staying fit is this: exercise is a lifestyle. And while for competitive athletes exercise and training pretty much dominate their waking hours, the amount of time they put in isn't the point. Rather, what I want to highlight is that exercise is a regular part of their lives. You and I can make fitness—regular exercise and a healthy diet—a regular part of our lives, too, even if we can only invest fifteen minutes each day in exercise. When exercise becomes as habitual as your morning cup of coffee, then you'll know you've adopted a fitness lifestyle.

Maintaining Motion

The overall goal of any osteoarthritis exercise program is to maintain motion, preserve strength, and decrease pain. Let me shorten that to a mantra for anyone suffering from osteoarthritis: motion is life. The muscle-building exercises outlined below are aimed at keeping your joints functioning as well as possible.

Arthritic inflammation of a joint can make it difficult to do even the seemingly simplest of tasks, such as reaching for a book or climbing the stairs. The temptation is to avoid any motions that cause pain, but the price is a heavy one to pay. When you do not use the complete range of motion of your joints, they can become stiff with contractures, which leads to additional loss in joint mobility and an increase in joint weakness—in other words, a never-ending cycle.

To keep all of your joints supple, stretched out, and strengthened, the major muscle groups around all of the joints must be exercised, with particular attention to the arthritic joints. An optimal osteoarthritis exercise regimen incorporates three types of strengthening exercises:

1. *Isometric* exercises, which tighten and strengthen specific muscles around a joint without moving the joint

2. *Isotonic* exercises, which involve moving the joint in contractions with a set amount of resistance

3. *Isokinetic* exercises, which contract the muscles at a specific speed with varying resistance

These basic exercise principles are the same ones we use in the USC Keck School of Medicine's Department of Orthopedic Surgery and in the training room for USC athletes, especially those who have been sidelined by illness or injury and must regain their athletic ability through a muscle-strengthening regimen.

A few words about stretching before we start. Whether you should stretch before an exercise workout continues to be a topic of hot debate in the sports medicine and fitness community. Not too long ago, it was a given: before you took an aerobics class, a bike ride, or a jog, you stretched to "warm up" the muscles to avoid injuries. But when experts at the CDC combed through more than a hundred papers looking at stretching studies, they found that people who stretched before exercise were no less likely to suffer injuries such as a pulled muscle. Indeed, some studies even indicated that stretching increased the chances for injury by straining the muscles at a vulnerable time: right before they were used in an extended physical workout.

Still, stretching does appear to achieve the goal of increased flexibility around joints. Perhaps the apparent failure of stretching to prevent injury occurs because the timing is wrong. It's not a matter of if but when to stretch. In other words, yes, you should stretch to keep your muscles, tendons, and ligaments flexible, but not necessarily before you do a fitness workout. Rather, think of stretching as something you do naturally throughout the day. Start when you first wake up and you're still in bed. Lying on your back, flex your hands and wiggle your fingers, your feet, and your toes. Then gently twist your body so that your bent legs are together facing in one direction and your arms in the other. Hold this body twist for ten seconds. Then switch sides and repeat. Return to lying on your back, and if you can, gently bring your folded legs, one at a time, to your chest and hold for ten seconds each. Finally, clasp your hands and raise them above your head to gently stretch your arms.

These are the kinds of gentle flexing exercises that you can do throughout the day, while you are sitting at a desk or watching TV. Think of stretching, then, not so much as exercise but as a normal part of your physically active lifestyle.

Isometric Exercises

As long as humans have been striving to stay fit, isometric exercises have been part of the regimen. Isometric exercise programs date back thousands of years. Certain static holds in the ancient physical arts of yoga and tai chi are examples of isometric exercise.

Isometrics were first brought to the modern public's attention in the early days of physical culture, the precursor to bodybuilding. Many of the great bodybuilders of the nineteenth century, notably Eugene Sandow, incorporated isometric exercises into their training regimes.

Isometrics are done in static positions. Pushing against a wall and holding the position is the classic example. Here are other popular isometric exercises.

UPPER BODY STRENGTHENING

- *Push-up.* Lie facedown on the ground with your arms spread outward like a T. Keep your legs fully extended and together. Put your hands flat on the ground just outside of your shoulder width. Push yourself up onto your hands and toes. Hold this position for at least ten seconds and then lower yourself to the ground. Repeat at least two times.

- *Lateral shoulder raise.* Stand with your feet shoulder width apart with your arms down at your sides. Raise your arms outward and upward until they are parallel with your shoulders. Hold this position for at least ten seconds. Repeat at least two times.

- *Superman.* Lie flat on your stomach with your arms pointed straight ahead, your legs fully extended, and the tops of your feet flat on the ground. Then lift your arms and legs off the ground; your midsection should remain on the ground. Keep your head and neck aligned with your torso. Hold this position for at least fifteen seconds. Repeat at least three times.

LOWER BODY STRENGTHENING

- *Squat.* Stand with your feet shoulder width apart and lower your body by bending your knees. Keep your torso upright and your hands out in front of you. When your knees are bent at a ninety-degree angle and your thighs are about parallel with the ground, stop and hold this position for at least ten seconds. Repeat at least two times.

- *Calf raise.* Stand with your feet inside of your shoulder width. Push up on your toes and the balls of your feet so that your calves are completely flexed. Hold this position for ten to fifteen seconds. Repeat two to four times.

- *Leg extension.* Sit on a chair with your torso upright and suck in your stomach muscles. Place your hands to your sides, knees bent and feet flat on the floor. Then lift both legs up until they are parallel to the floor. Hold this position for at least ten seconds. Repeat at least two times.

Isotonic Exercises

Isotonic exercise really came into its own with the advent of the modern-day bodybuilding culture in the 1950s at Muscle Beach in Venice, California. When the muscle carries a static weight over a specific range of motion, that's isotonic exercise. A biceps curl is a classic example where the muscle has to work against a set resistance through the range of motion.

Both free weights and machines can be used for isotonic exercises. You don't need a great deal of equipment: a few dumbbells and an exercise bench will do. This is also the perfect excuse to join the local Y or gym.

If you don't have access to weights, then you can perform resistance exercises with just the weight of your own body. Pull-ups, push-ups, crunches, squats, and lunges are all examples.

A compromise between working out with no equipment at all and getting a full gym membership is to use resistance bands. These giant rubber bands typically have handles on the ends. You can even increase the intensity and resistance by using two bands at once.

Here are some classic isotonic exercises.

- *Sissy squats.* These work the lower quadriceps. Hold on to a wall or bench for support and then rise up onto your toes and lean back very slightly. Still on your toes and with your back straight, sink slowly into a shallow squat. Repeat five to ten times.

- *Triceps press-ups.* In a sitting position on a bench (or armless chair) with your feet on the ground in front of you, face away from the bench and extend your legs in front of you. Place the palms of your hands on the bench. Raise and lower your body by straightening and bending your arms at the elbow. Repeat five times.

- *Push-ups.* These work the chest, shoulders, and biceps. Position your arms slightly wider than your shoulders, and then place your hands on an exercise bench or the floor and raise and lower your body by straightening and bending your arms. Repeat five times.

- *Partial sit-ups.* This exercise works the abdominals. Lie on the floor with your knees raised and place your hands behind your head. Keep your elbows pointing outward. Without pulling up on your head with your arms, raise your shoulders up from the ground and then lower them back down. Repeat five times.

- *Oblique sit-ups.* To work the abdominals and obliques, repeat the partial sit-ups described in the preceding exercise, but cross one leg over the other, resting the right foot on the left knee. Raise your shoulders and while twisting from the waist, touch your right elbow to your left knee. Repeat five times and then switch sides.

Isokinetic Exercises

In this type of exercise, the speed of muscle contractions remains unchanged regardless of how much effort is exerted. Isokinetic exercise is all about variable resistance, achieved with the help of a machine. With a preset speed of contraction, muscles and joints will be allowed their full range of motion without the risk of injury.

Isokinetic exercise first surfaced with the fitness boom of the 1980s and the advent of modern (and now digitally controlled) exercise equipment. This type of exercise minimizes the risk of injury by ensuring that the force opposing the movement is not greater than the force the muscles can exert. It also allows for a specific range of movements to be targeted much more precisely than is possible with isometric exercises.

To do an isokinetic exercise properly, you really need a machine that sets a constant speed of motion, such as those made by manufacturers Cybex and Biodex. You'll find equipment by both brands at most gyms these days.

Aerobic Exercise with Hydro Power

In this chapter, we've focused on strength-building exercise. But as we discussed in Chapter 3, aerobic exercise is equally important because it increases your overall heart rate and cardiovascular fitness. With increased muscular strength, arthritic patients have a better mental attitude and experience improvement in their arthritis symptoms. As previously noted, before you undertake any program of aerobic exercise, consider any potential heart problems or other medical conditions, as well as the limitations imposed by painful arthritic joints.

Walking at a brisk pace may be the perfect aerobic exercise. It's relatively low impact, it requires no special equipment except a good pair of walking shoes, and you don't need any training. Because we do it naturally, my patients are sometimes incredulous that walking even counts as exercise. Remember, the overall goal of any osteoarthritis exercise program is to maintain motion, and walking is the human body's most natural form of motion.

But let's say that even walking is difficult for you, or you just want to mix up your landlocked fitness program with a little splash of fun. Fortunately, water workouts have never been so diverse. If you want a new way to get a cardiac workout, consider Aqua Zumba, a spin-off of the popular cardio craze. Similarly, high-powered aqua kickboxing, which combines martial arts, athletic drills, and plyometric jumps, provides an excellent cross-training workout. In both programs, water rather than weights provides the resistance, and you can move at your own pace.

If you've tried yoga but find the static positions hard to maintain, then consider water yoga. As with regular yoga, classes differ in degrees of difficulty, but the buoyancy water provides protects your joints, while its resistance loads your muscles.

Cycling is excellent for hip strengthening, but if you're wary of the road and the stationary bike leaves you bored, then your ship has arrived: the hydrobike. Instead of pedaling in a gym or in your living room, with a hydrobike you are gliding across a picturesque waterway. Many resort communities with a beach or lake offer this latest exercise gadget, which is equal parts fun and fitness.

The Four Guiding Principles of OA Exercise

Exercise must be performed on a consistent basis if it's going to provide benefits. Whatever exercise and fitness regimen you choose, follow these guidelines:

1. *Be consistent.* Exercises should be done daily according to an individualized program.

2. *Build up gradually.* Start with easier exercises through lesser ranges of motion and slowly increase both resistance and range of motion.

3. *Exercise when you are less symptomatic.* Sometimes arthritis patients have more stiffness and pain in the morning. Find the time of day when your joints are most comfortable and exercise then.

4. *Set manageable goals.* A six-month "master plan" to change your life can seem daunting. Instead, start with a small commitment—say, three weeks of walking twenty minutes a day—and see how it goes.

There is no fixed ideal as to how much and how often you should do the exercises in your routine. But here's a general rule of thumb: let pain be your guide and do not do too much exercise too fast. Pay attention to how you feel during your workout. If you feel excessive pain or if your joints are swollen and warm, modify your activity until the pain and swelling subside.

KEEPING YOUR GAIT STRAIGHT

As discussed in Chapter 3, it is important that people with osteoarthritis exercise in a controlled fashion under the supervision of a physical or occupational therapist. An exercise program that is too vigorous can harm your joints, even if your primary form of exercise is walking. You may not realize it, but your gait—how you walk or run—can unnecessarily increase the load on your knee and hip joints and increase your chances of developing arthritis.

Trained physical therapists—you will find them practicing in hospitals or other clinical settings—can watch your gait and observe how your feet, knees, and hips work together. Many physical therapists use video cameras so you can see for yourself what the problem is.

I want to underscore that the hips are key to proper gait. Too often, conventional sports medicine or physical therapy focuses just on how the feet and knees work together. However, my USC colleague Chris Powers, codirector of the Musculoskeletal Biomechanics Research Lab, has an ongoing study that already has produced fascinating results. He concludes that for amateur, collegiate, and professional athletes, the usefulness of hip strengthening in avoiding injury has been vastly underrated. "Strength training is not enough; you have to move well," he says, and the hips are equally important in moving well, as are the knees.

Exercises to strengthen the hips are leg lifts, squats, and lunges. Cycling (including both traditional upright or stationary bikes and recumbent bikes) provides strengthening of the entire hip without impact.

Diet

At the outset of the book, I made the commitment to you that I would be perfectly honest when it comes to what science has to say about arthritis treatment. Here are the facts, based on our current knowledge, regarding diet: there is no compelling evidence that there is any "best" diet. No diet has been proven to either improve your osteoarthritis or make it worse.

Yes, adopting a diet that promotes a healthy weight is extremely beneficial. As discussed in Chapter 3, obesity is a huge contributing factor to the rising number of osteoarthritis sufferers, because of the excess load exerted on the joints (particularly the knees) by extra weight and because obesity (especially excessive belly fat) promotes inflammation that probably degrades cartilage.

Finding Your Food Muse

Arriving at your optimal weight is a very individualized process, influenced by what foods you like and by your body chemistry. You have to find your own food muse. And when you do, you must incorporate it into your fitness lifestyle, which, as we talked about earlier, also includes exercise.

Marilyn Monroe did. In the recent barrage of media coverage on the fiftieth anniversary of the death of Hollywood's most iconic actress, one item really caught my eye. The London *Daily Mail* published an article about her diet, and I'm betting that in a hundred years you could never guess what she ate to maintain her perfectly voluptuous figure. In an interview published shortly before her death, the sex goddess laid out her daily diet and fitness regimen. She said she began her day with a "slimming" breakfast of two raw eggs in warm milk. For lunch, she had broiled steak, liver, or lamb chops with a handful of carrots. Supper usually consisted of a hot fudge sundae and nothing else. To stay toned, she worked out for ten minutes a day with a variety of isometric exercises. "I couldn't stand exercise if I had to feel regimented about it," said the blond bombshell.

No, I'm not advocating here that everyone adopt the Marilyn Monroe diet and fitness plan and eat only hot fudge sundaes for dinner. As tempting as her eating habits might have been, we'll never know what Marilyn would have looked like in middle age had she maintained that, um, very individualistic diet. Rather, let's give the lady a posthumous round of applause for incorporating into her lifestyle a diet and exercise regimen that worked for her.

In Praise of the "Anti-Inflammatory Diet"

Now, you may be wondering, what do I eat? I follow a diet high in whole grains and fresh fruits and vegetables and low in animal protein (including dairy), salt, and sugar. You might call it a semi-vegan (or vegan adjacent) diet. I never have red meat and I avoid chicken, lamb, and pork. I rarely eat eggs and seafood, and I get protein from beans, nuts, and soy-based sources such as tofu and tempeh. I strive to eat organic foods to avoid hormonal additives and pesticides.

Kind of makes me a health nut, right? You might ask why I bother, since, as I mentioned before, there's no compelling evidence that any particular diet either improves osteoarthritis or makes it worse. I have two answers. First, I eat as I do for my overall fitness—that is, to maintain my proper weight and to avoid chronic health issues such as heart disease, stroke, hypertension, diabetes, and cancer. Almost everything I read supports this.

Second, while there's no cold hard science proving that the diet I eat will help me to avoid chronic diseases, including osteoarthritis, there are many scientific studies *indicating* that my type of diet lowers the body's "inflammatory thermostat." Conversely, there's a growing body of evidence that a diet high in red and processed meats and high in fat, sugar, salt, and simple carbs such as those in white bread and packaged sweets (cookies, cakes, pastries) is pro-inflammatory. So, all things considered, I'll take my chances with the less inflammatory diet as I await further scientific clarification.

At this moment, the science of diet and nutrition cannot be more definitive as to which foods play a helpful or harmful role in osteoarthritis. Why? Because most nutritional studies are conducted on lab animals. Useful information can be gleaned from these animal studies (enough to convince me, for example, that I'm on the right diet pathway), but ultimately they're inherently limited by the fact that a rat, a rabbit, or a rhesus monkey isn't a human being and responds differently to foods than you or I do.

There's no such thing as a one-size-fits-all diet plan. Ultimately, we're all different, and each of us has to find the diet that works best for us—helping us to achieve and maintain our proper weight while delivering the nutrients we need. My anti-inflammatory, semi-vegan diet works for me. With it I can maintain a proper weight without too much effort, and generally I feel better than I did on the high-animal-protein diet that I ate for decades.

How can you find your food muse, other than trial and error? I have two books to recommend, both authored by scientific and medical professionals. *The L.A. Shape Diet,* by David Heber, MD, PhD, is designed to create a personalized diet plan that fits with your body type. For those who want to embrace a more plant-based diet, then I recommend *The China Study,* by Cornell University professor T. Colin Campbell, PhD, and his son Thomas M. Campbell, MD.

Takeaways

In this chapter we learned that diet and exercise, when incorporated into an overall lifestyle, can play important roles in improving the quality of life if you suffer from osteoarthritis. Strength-building exercises that facilitate the movements of the joints should be part of any osteoarthritis exercise regimen. Use low-impact aerobic exercises such as walking and "hydro sports" to maintain proper weight and build overall cardiovascular health. Scientific studies indicate that an anti-inflammatory, plant-protein-based diet can contribute to overall health, although there is no definitive evidence that any specific kind of diet, or eating or avoiding any particular foods or food groups, prevents arthritis or promotes it.

6

DIAGNOSTICS AND SURGERY

Do you remember the lyrics to an antiwar song by Edwin Starr that was the number one hit in America for three weeks in 1970? They went like this: "War. Huh! What is it good for? Absolutely nothing." Actually, the Vietnam War, not to mention World Wars I and II, were good for orthopedic surgery. Modern orthopedics was developed on battlefields of the twentieth century by surgeons who had a virtually unlimited supply of young men with broken bones, severed muscles, and torn ligaments and tendons to try different techniques on.

Traction and splinting were developed during World War I. The use of intramedullary rods (a metal rod forced into the cavity of a bone) to treat fractures of the femur was developed by German field surgeons during World War II. Traction was the standard method of treating thigh bone fractures until the late 1970s, when external fixation of fractures (which had been refined by American military surgeons during the Vietnam War) became widespread.

But while orthopedics can be said to have come of age because of modern-day warfare, prior to that orthopedics was largely focused on crippled children. The first orthopedic institute, a hospital dedicated to the treatment of children's skeletal deformities, was established by

Jean-André Venel in France. (In fact, the term *orthopedics* itself refers to children, as it is derived from the Greek *orthos,* "correct, straight," and *paideion,* "child," and was coined by another French surgeon, Nicolas Andry, in 1741 when he published *Orthopaedia, or the Art of Correcting and Preventing Deformities in Children.*)

Today, orthopedics is the branch of medicine concerned with the diagnosis, treatment, rehabilitation, and prevention of injuries and diseases of the body's musculoskeletal system, including bones, joints, ligaments, tendons, muscles, and nerves.

In this chapter, I will tell you step by step what to expect when you and your doctor have decided that surgical intervention is the best option for treating an arthritic condition. While we'll focus on conventional surgical procedures—what is available in the here and now—let me say that I have seen remarkable advances in orthopedic surgery during the thirty years that I've been in the operating room. Technological innovations in equipment have revolutionized the field. Trimming meniscus tears today is an outpatient procedure done with arthroscopic equipment and takes one-fifth of the time it used to; previously, the entire meniscus had to be removed, and the patient had to stay in the hospital for up to two days. Now I can reconstruct a dislocated shoulder and torn ligament with three small incisions in a forty-five-minute outpatient procedure that heals in days; no longer do I need to admit the patient to the hospital for a full-on open shoulder incision and weeks of recovery time. So compared to the Middle Ages, when broken limbs were slathered with horse's blood that was allowed to dry into a makeshift cast, this is a good time to be a patient with an orthopedic ailment.

When Surgery Feels Right

Most of my patients know when surgery feels like the right option. Their joints become stiff and swollen, and soon they come to realize that simple everyday activities—getting out of the car, climbing a staircase— are suddenly onerous tasks. The different forms of arthritis can have a multitude of symptoms and involve a variety of organs. Fortunately, osteoarthritis usually involves a few joints, or just one, and is clearly different from the inflammatory types of arthritis.

Depending on their insurance plan, the patients I see often have gone first to their internist or family practitioner, who is most familiar with their medical history. More recently, patients whose health plan allows them to go directly to specialists who deal with joint pain, whether it's an orthopedic surgeon like me or a rheumatologist.

What's the difference? Orthopedic surgeons deal with muscles, joints, and bone problems; we use both surgical and nonsurgical treatment plans. A rheumatologist is fully trained in general internal medicine with an additional two years of training focusing solely on the rare arthritic diseases. These doctors can diagnose and treat arthritis with nonsurgical techniques.

Patients with serious and extensive problems generally need to have further testing and in-depth evaluations beyond what the average generalist does. Patients can always call their local county medical society or any local branch of the Arthritis Foundation for referrals to appropriate, well-trained physicians. It is important that the patient have a good relationship with the doctor, as arthritis is a chronic disease and the patient will be under the doctor's care for many years.

BETTER SEX AFTER SURGERY

The idea that orthopedic surgery can promote better sex might be counterintuitive. But just ask Louise.

Louise is a lovely sixty-one-year-old woman who knew it was time for hip replacement surgery. I actually explored a variety of alternatives that could temporarily relieve the pain she was suffering, but she was determined. "Dr. Vangsness, I want my love life back, and I don't want just a one-night stand," she told me unabashedly. I scheduled surgery for her with a colleague the following week.

(Continues)

BETTER SEX AFTER SURGERY (Continued)

She was typical of many of my patients—male and female—who suffer pain from arthritic joints when fooling around with their significant other. Having sex is not much fun when you have grinding pain with every bump and grind. The discomfort from an arthritic hip, knee, or neck can be enough to throw a wet blanket on even the most enthusiastic Romeo or Juliet.

If you wonder if Louise isn't a bit young to have hip replacement surgery, let me set the record straight. Much of the increase in hip surgery has been fueled by the middle-aged, those between the ages of forty-five and sixty-five. In that age group, hip replacements nearly tripled, to 128,000, during the past decade.

There is an orthopedic surgeon who has created a website, complete with illustrations, showing safer positions for sexual activity after hip replacement surgery. Find it at http://ortho chick.squarespace.com/sex-after-joint-replacement.

Assessing Medical History and Condition

During your first visit, the doctor will review your medical problems and get an understanding of your current lifestyle and its limitations. Certain forms of arthritis appear to run in families, and a history of your parents and siblings can be relevant. Your physician will focus on your main complaints and any symptoms associated with them.

As we've seen, symptoms for arthritis can vary tremendously, from weight loss and fever to involvement of the spine or skin. Often, asking questions about all the major organ symptoms can help a doctor make a specific arthritis diagnosis. Fortunately, most forms of osteoarthritis are usually localized to one joint.

During a simple walking demonstration, the physician will view your gait, paying particular attention to the mobility at the hip and knee joints. Range of motion of all joints will be tested to see if motion is symmetrical on the left and right. At that time, each joint can be examined for warmth, redness, or swelling—the characteristic signs of arthritis. With more extensive involvement, joints can become deformed, and this is very evident on exam. Examination for nodules and rashes is important, as many rare forms of arthritis can affect the skin.

Getting the Right Diagnosis

There are many great medical achievements of the modern era. For orthopedic doctors, hands down, it's the invention of the X-ray machine, the device that has been used as the standard device for examinations of bones beginning in 1896.

As they were more than a hundred years ago, X-rays are the critical diagnostic tools for evaluating joint pathology. With osteoarthritis, the joint space becomes narrowed as the articular surface is worn away. Regular wear and tear can cause erosions and deformations of the ends of the joint. Bone tissue is continually active, and the bone's reaction to arthritis can result in the formation of peripheral bony growth deposits called spurs, in which normally round joints become flattened. Bone ends can become abnormally dense and hard, a condition known as sclerosis. All of these are visible in X-rays.

In joints afflicted by inflammatory arthritis, especially rheumatoid arthritis, there is a symmetrical narrowing of the joint, as opposed to the irregular wearing away of the articular cartilage seen with osteoarthritis. There is also loss of bone density around the joint in RA, with swelling in the tissue surrounding the joint.

X-rays are also important for evaluating the initial status of the joint so that it may be followed over time. If surgery is being contemplated, decisions about the type of surgery can be made after viewing the X-rays.

Certain other diseases, such as ankylosing spondylitis, produce characteristic changes in the spine that can be seen easily on X-ray. These changes are called "bamboo spine." Occasionally, radio-opaque dye may be inserted into a joint to give contrast to the joint line as well as locate other parts of the joint, such as the meniscus in the knee or the labrum in the hip. More sophisticated tests such as magnetic resonance imaging (MRI) or CT scans can be used to help diagnose the status of the joint.

Tests, Tests, and More Tests

Besides X-rays, the other critical diagnostic tool in determining whether surgery is necessary is lab tests. Most of these tests can be completed in a single trip to a doctor, with the results available within days. These tests, in combination with the patient's history and physical exam, will help the experienced physician accurately understand the arthritis diagnosis.

Blood Tests

If blood tests are required, your physician will first take a sample of your blood for a complete blood count. Blood consists of specific cell types, such as red blood cells, white blood cells, and platelets, immersed in a colorless fluid called plasma. A complete blood count, or CBC, is a very nonspecific test that gives the physician a picture of the patient's overall health. Also, it can help the doctor narrow down the possible diagnosis. For example, the process of inflammation can cause many different changes to the patient's blood count. The white count can go up, the platelet count can go up, and the red cell blood count can go down, signaling anemia. The white cell count can increase from any infection, so a careful medical history and physical exam should help determine the importance of an elevated white blood count.

Another nonspecific test is a chemical profile. The blood plasma contains many proteins and other substances. Common proteins we look for include antibodies, clotting factors, and various enzymes. For instance, kidney function can be measured by following creatinine levels. An elevation in the level of uric acid can indicate gout.

Other tests are more specific. Thyroid tests can establish the activity level of the thyroid, which can aggravate signs and symptoms of the rarer types of arthritis. The sedimentation profile (also known as the sed rate) is a simple measure of inflammation occurring throughout the body: the sedimentation rate is high in most types of inflammatory arthritis but usually near normal in osteoarthritis.

Approximately 80 percent of patients with rheumatoid arthritis have RF (an autoantibody) in their blood, and the concentration of RF is used as an indicator of the disease, with a higher concentration implying more severe rheumatoid arthritis. Some scientists think that RF causes the disease, while others think it is the body's response to the inflammation associated with the disease. Sometimes it takes months for the RF to show up in the blood, and some people have all the symptoms of RA but do not have this factor in their blood; these people are called seronegative. An abnormal level of RF can also occur as a result of inflammatory infectious disease other than RA, adding further to the confusion. In any event, the RF test is the best tool we have for diagnosing RA at this time. The citrullinated peptide (CCP) antibody blood test also confirms rheumatoid arthritis.

Urinalysis

Examination of the urine is valuable for evaluating kidney function. Looking for different chemicals and particular proteins or blood can help the doctor determine if there are problems with the kidneys.

Antinuclear Antibody (ANA)

The antinuclear antibody (ANA) is an abnormal protein found in the blood. Some laboratories call the test for ANA the fluorescent antibody nuclear test (FANA), as they use fluorescent dye to help identify these antibodies.

This test is the best we have at the present time to look for lupus (SLE), although additional testing will be needed to establish whether that disease is present. However, it is important to understand that patients with other diseases can have positive ANA tests. For example, about 50 percent of RA patients test positive.

It is interesting that approximately 5 percent of elderly patients can have both positive RF and positive ANA tests without having a disease; the reason for this is uncertain.

Other tests that may be used in an effort to diagnose lupus are the LE test (though this is not commonly used these days) and the serum complement test. The latter is also used to monitor disease activity once lupus has been diagnosed.

Joint Fluid Tests

Synovial fluid in a healthy joint is clear and thick, and is often described as "stringy." If a joint is affected by an inflammatory or infectious process, the synovial fluid can become cloudy and puslike. Doctors will often "tap" a joint by inserting a sterile needle and removing fluid for visual and chemical analysis. This fluid can be visualized with a special dye called a gram stain and/or cultured to confirm the presence of infectious bacteria. A cell count can be made to determine the number and types of white blood cells in the joint fluid, as joint inflammation can be confirmed by a high white blood cell count. The fluid can be examined under a specialized polarized microscope for crystals, the presence of which confirms the presence of gout or pseudogout.

Surgical Options

The overall treatment plan for degenerative arthritis involves addressing the pain from joints. This is really about controlling the ongoing inflammation process. If conservative nonsurgical treatments such as physical therapy, medications, and weight loss fail to relieve the pain of arthritis, patients currently have no real alternative other than surgery. Think of surgery less as a last resort and more as another option for treatment. After all, if you cannot enjoy your everyday life and are forced to sit on the sidelines, debilitated by pain and immobility, then surgery can be a godsend.

Many different surgical procedures are designed to alleviate the pain, slow down or prevent ongoing cartilage damage, and at the same time restore joint stability and mobility for everyday use. Of particular concern is excessive joint pain at night, such that your sleep is interrupted. These are all criteria that demonstrate a decrease in the quality of life and perhaps suggest the need for surgical intervention.

All operations involve risk; therefore, you and your doctor need to discuss the best options. Different types of surgical procedures can be used to treat arthritic joints. The exact procedure for you will depend on your age, the joint involved, associated pathologies about the joint, alignment of the joint, and individual needs.

Arthroscopy

In the last two decades developments in arthroscopic surgery have resulted in a tremendous improvement in the treatment of joint pain. An arthroscope is an instrument in which bundles of transparent fibers transmit light into the joint through an instrument about the diameter of a straw. Images are transmitted back to a high-definition flat-screen monitor in the operating suite, which allows the surgeon to visualize and evaluate the entire inside of the joint, including the articular surfaces and various soft tissues, through two or three small incisions, called portals. Following the procedure, the portals, which are only a few millimeters in diameter, are sutured closed. This is a very straightforward surgery performed as an outpatient procedure.

Small tools including tiny scalpels, shaving instruments, and grabbing and rasping (smoothing) instruments are used to inspect or operate on any joint. The surgeon can trim articular cartilage surface edges that have separated from the bone, like paint peeling from the ceiling or linoleum peeling from the floor; removing these areas of useless, malfunctioning tissue can provide pain relief. Often articular cartilage can break off and fall into the joint, creating a painful loose body floating around. These bodies can be easily removed with a tiny suction tube. Smoothing rough surfaces and trimming bone spurs often can help relieve arthritis pain. However, there is no absolute guarantee that smoothing down or shaving areas of degenerative arthritis will give long-term relief. The best results usually occur when a patient clearly has strong mechanical symptoms (such as locking or catching).

Overall, the outcome from arthroscopic surgery for osteoarthritis is very different for each patient. However, generally there is a low health risk with a high pain relief benefit.

Synovectomy

Joints can become very inflamed due to the ongoing process of osteoarthritis, as discussed earlier. Some inflammatory arthritis conditions, most commonly rheumatoid arthritis, can create a painful, inflamed synovium, the tissue lining the joint. Removing this lining in a procedure called a synovectomy can reduce pain and swelling and potentially prevent or delay ongoing destruction of the cartilage and bone. Synovectomy can be done as an open procedure or through arthroscopic techniques. However, the synovium can regrow; therefore there can be no guarantee.

Osteotomy

Osteotomy is a surgical procedure to restore the proper mechanical axis of a joint—essentially a realignment. This can change the motion of the joint, shifting the load-bearing articular cartilage surfaces to a less painful and perhaps healthier area of the joint. The bones are cut, moved into their new alignment, and held in place with plates and screws. It is commonly done in the lower extremity about the knee to correct curvature of either the femur or the tibia, which can increase wear and tear on the knee joint.

There is no certain relief of pain with this surgery, and an osteotomy does carry health risks for the patient. It also requires a short hospital stay. Having the procedure can be compared to rotating the tires on your car in an attempt to extend the wear of the tires. The surgery should relieve pain in the short term, but over the long term the joint continues to degenerate.

Resection

Occasionally a surgeon can actually remove a part of the end of a bone that has been damaged by osteoarthritis. In theory, removing this damaged part will provide the patient with pain relief. This surgery is usually performed in certain areas of the body, such as the acromioclavicular joint (in the shoulder) or on the ends of the metatarsals (the bones in the toes). Resection can also be performed in the wrists and the hands.

Cartilage Transplantation

Three bones meet within the knee joint: the femur (the thigh bone), the tibia (the shin bone), and the patella (the kneecap). As in many other joints, the surfaces of these bones are covered where they meet with a durable slick lining called articular cartilage. This type of cartilage has unique biochemical and physical qualities that make it nearly frictionless—when functioning properly, articular cartilage has less friction than two pieces of ice sliding on each other. But what makes articular cartilage uniquely smooth—its lack of nerve and blood supply—also means that it has a very limited capacity for self-repair. Worse, shallow damage often does not trigger pain, so a person whose joint has suffered minor damage may not even know it, and may engage in activities that worsen the damage. Plus an articular cartilage defect that starts out small still has the potential to have a physical and chemical domino effect on the surrounding normal articular cartilage.

Researchers have been trying to grow artificial articular cartilage that could be inserted into a diseased joint. A number of tissue engineering materials are currently being investigated, but to date no one has grown true articular cartilage. So surgeons fill these "potholes" in the cartilage with graft materials. We'll explore further the directions science is taking in this area later in the book.

Currently, a cartilage transplant procedure can be performed where there is focal cartilage damage—small areas that were once normal joint surface but currently have damaged articular cartilage. In this transplant procedure, which is most commonly performed on the knee, small pieces of cartilage with their underlying bone are taken from other parts of the knee (autografts), or larger grafts can be taken from a registered national tissue bank, and are screwed, pinned, wedged, or glued in place in the damaged area. It takes a minimum of two months for this transplanted cartilage and bone composite to heal; many times a patient will use crutches during this period. There is very little problem with tissue rejection, as there is such a low blood supply to these tissues. Here too, the idea is to give pain relief in an effort to delay another surgery, such as a future total knee replacement.

Yet another cartilage transplant procedure involves having your own cartilage grown in a lab and reinserting it into small focal defects in the body. This is generally done about the knee, but occasionally is done around the ankle, hip, or shoulder. During an arthroscopy, the surgeon can see whether there is a small area of cartilage degeneration that is exposing the underlying bone. The surgeon then can take a pea-sized sample of cartilage from a non-weight-bearing area and send it to a lab, Genzyme Biology in Boston, where the cells are incubated and allowed to reproduce. In as little as three weeks, the newly grown cartilage will be ready to be reimplanted in a second procedure in which the knee is opened, the edges of the defect are trimmed, and a patch of periosteum (tissue surrounding the bone) is harvested, sewn over the bed, and then sealed with a tissue glue. The newly cultured cells—called an autologous chondrocyte implant (ACI)—can then be injected under this patch. Long-term follow-up studies of up to ten years have shown that ACIs produce good-quality articular cartilage and pain relief. Refinements are constantly being introduced, and this surgery is rapidly evolving into an arthroscopic procedure with different scaffolds (materials to hold cells) and cell combinatins. There are many research endeavors in this field of "pothole filling" around the world.

Joint Fusion

Occasionally an arthrodesis (fusion) may be recommended. This is an operative procedure to fuse the joint in an effort to reduce pain and improve stability. With a fusion, the joint has no ability to move and flex, yet pain can be markedly reduced. This is commonly done with the spine, foot, ankle, and wrist. Much more rarely it is performed in the knee, the shoulder, or the hip. Arthrodesis of the hips and knees (rare) can be done in the face of infection or in patients who are too young to have artificial joints. The procedure involves cutting out the ends of the bones and putting a bone graft in this area, then binding them together with plates or screws.

Arthroplasty

An arthroplasty is a procedure where both ends of the damaged joint are removed and replaced with a plastic-and-metal or ceramic implant. Hips and knees are the most commonly replaced joint, but shoulders, fingers, elbows, and ankles can also undergo arthroplasty. We can also now replace parts of the knee (partial replacements) to avoid having to remove the entire natural joint; this can be done in the shoulder and hip as well. Sometimes this is preferred over total joint replacement, for if and when a partial replacement fails, the patient can always undergo a total joint replacement.

The purpose of this more involved operation is pain relief with restoration of a good amount of function. Patients can never be promised full function after joint replacement, but they will be able to perform many activities of daily living. Sleep and activities including stair climbing are remarkably improved with arthroplasty in the knees and hips. Many of my patients find that their overall quality of life is demonstrably improved following a joint replacement. The government recognizes joint replacement surgery as having some of the best outcomes in medicine.

The first American total joint and hip replacement procedures were performed in the 1960s. Now there are hundreds of thousands of joint reconstructions performed every year. Joint replacement generally requires a hospital admission for three to five days, and it is commonly done in association with a blood transfusion. While complications can arise, they are generally uncommon (less than 1–2 percent of cases).

Common complications are blood clots, loosening of the prosthesis, dislocation of the prosthesis, and wearing down of the components of the plastic or metal over time. Debris caused by wear can result in an inflammatory reaction, which over a long period of time can loosen the joint. Infections are serious complications that occur in about one-half of 1 percent of these surgeries. Administering prophylactic antibiotics prior to surgery and after surgery, along with strict sterile techniques, helps to minimize infection.

Surgery Issues: Anesthesia to Insurance

You can never ask too many questions when it comes to a surgical procedure. The problem for most patients is knowing which questions to ask. Before you undergo surgery, all your questions should be answered and you and your doctor should discuss your expectations.

Here are issues every patient should address before going under the knife.

Surgery Risks

Risks of surgery include infection, blood clots, thrombophlebitis, ongoing joint pain, stiffness, and nerve or blood vessel damage, as well as the risks of anesthesia. It is important that you discuss with your surgeon the risks and benefits of the surgery as it applies to you and your lifestyle.

Selecting a Surgeon

Your personal physician can point you to a surgeon, usually an orthopedic surgeon, who has specialized training and experience in surgical joint procedures. As previously noted, orthopedic surgeons perform operations involving the musculoskeletal system, including joints, muscles, and bones. The orthopedic surgeon should be board certified, which establishes that he or she has completed the required five years of training after medical school (plus, commonly, a fellowship, which is an additional year of training in various specific areas) and has passed an examination documenting his or her knowledge. As an academic surgeon, I did two fellowships. It is very easy to research your surgeon's educational background and credentials on the internet.

Second Opinion

I am always in favor of second opinions, and if you request the names of other doctors who can provide a second opinion, a surgeon should provide a short list. Your referring physician can also help with this, or you can contact the local medical society.

Selecting a Hospital

The right hospital is very important for the success of any surgery. A surgeon generally works out of a specific hospital, so it's important that the hospital have an excellent record and reputation, as its staff will be preparing you for surgery and caring for you afterward. Physical therapy and occupational therapy are paramount in the immediate postoperative time at the hospital, so include this in your assessment. Look for a medical center with strong orthopedic surgeons and rheumatologists, as well as internal medicine doctors, cardiologists, and infectious disease specialists in case there are any complications. Depending on your individual insurance plan and your doctor's preferences, the hospital you go to may not be close to your home. Many orthopedic surgeons perform certain operations as outpatient procedures in a certified surgery center.

Anesthesia

Anesthesia has undergone great developments in the last couple of decades. An anesthesiologist or nurse anesthetist will meet you before the surgery and will be present during your entire operation to monitor your breathing and blood pressure. Generally there are three types of anesthesia that can be used in surgery:

- *General anesthesia.* Sleep-inducing medicine is administered, and you are attached to a respirator that continues to deliver oxygen to your body. This procedure requires close monitoring.

- *Spinal or regional anesthesia.* Here the anesthesia is injected into the spinal canal or adjacent to the spinal canal, interrupting the nerve sensation down the legs or up the arms. These are generally used for hip, knee, or other lower-extremity surgery.

- *Nerve blocks.* This regional anesthesia involves instilling an anesthetic right near a specific series of nerves involved with the area of the extremity that will be operated upon. These nerve blocks are commonly used for shoulder, elbow, and hand surgery or for foot surgery. A small external pain pump is now sometimes used to continuously deliver anesthesia through a small tube positioned under the skin adjacent to the nerve. This can be left in place for several days for pain control while the patient is recovering at home.

Insurance Evaluation

It is important that you understand your health care plan and the benefits that are offered. It's important to look at what the plan provides in terms of medications after surgery; physical therapy, either at home or at the hospital; assistive devices for use around the house, such as crutches, a raised toilet seat, and grip bars for toilet and tub; and the possibility of a home health care provider or a private-duty nurse. The internet has developed into a great tool for the consumer for this.

Preoperative Evaluation

If you are older than fifty, your orthopedic surgeon may have you see an internist, a family practitioner, or a primary care physician to complete a medical examination emphasizing heart, lung, and kidney function to make sure that you can safely undergo a general anesthetic. Younger patients who are healthy really only need simple blood tests prior to surgery.

Preoperative Arrangements

A discussion with your doctor and a nurse about considerations for your return home is imperative. This includes driving as well as simple activities of living such as stair climbing, getting in and out of a chair, and bathing. Eating arrangements such as shopping and cooking should be made prior to surgery. You may want to adjust your home to accommodate transitional sleeping arrangements if bedroom access is not convenient. Arranging for people to help you during the first few weeks after surgery may be very useful. Be familiar with whether you will be using crutches, a cane, or perhaps a walker after surgery and how this will affect you at your home and during physical therapy. A short-term handicap placard can be issued for driving. Many hospitals offer preoperative classes to prepare you for surgery.

Further, you should make sure to discuss recovery time and get a rough estimate of how long it will be before you can return to various activities of daily living and when you can begin a physical therapy regimen. Follow-up doctor's appointments and physical therapy appointments should be arranged prior to surgery.

When you pack for a hospital stay, include items such as slippers, toothbrush, glasses, bathrobe, reading matter, and other personal items.

Takeaways

Modern-day orthopedics was developed on the battlefields of the twentieth century, where field surgeons originated many of the procedures that still dominate orthopedics in the twenty-first century. The wide use of arthroscopic surgical procedures beginning in the 1970s, using miniature instruments and video monitors, revolutionized orthopedics by reducing the risk of infection and shortening recovery time.

Getting the right diagnosis for your specific arthritic condition is imperative, as it will determine not only which surgical procedure is best but whether surgery is necessary at all.

Finally, preparation for surgery should not simply be left up to your doctor, no matter how good he or she is. Use the various sections of this chapter to research and prepare for the full range of issues that can emerge before and after surgery.

7

DRUGS OF MANY CHOICES

In the beginning, there was aspirin. Hippocrates wrote about the therapeutic use of tea made from the bark of the European white willow tree—the original source of salicylic acid, a principal ingredient in what we now call aspirin—for treating inflamed joints. And then . . . well, that was about it when it came to the pharmacological treatment of osteoarthritis for, oh, the next couple of millennia. Seriously. Salicylic acid was the original and only wonder drug for most of recorded history, and Hippocrates would have made a killing if he could have patented willow bark tea.

The nineteenth century saw the active ingredient in willow bark isolated and then modified to a less toxic version that the Bayer company branded "aspirin." Even today, venerable aspirin, in its various time-release and buffered forms, remains a staple in the treatment of osteoarthritis.

Aspirin's popularity declined with the first breakthrough of modern pharmacology and the development of acetaminophen (Tylenol) in 1956 and the next generation of non-narcotic, nonsteroidal anti-inflammatory analgesic (painkilling) drugs usually abbreviated NSAIDs and pronounced "en-saids", notably ibuprofen (Advil, Motrin) in 1962, naproxen (Aleve) in 1976, and COX-2 inhibitors (Celebrex) in 1999.

They all offered pain relief with less of the stomach irritation that high doses of aspirin could have.

In this chapter, we'll discuss the pharmacological remedies available for osteoarthritis pain and inflammation. Some of the products are available over the counter, but our focus in this chapter is on drugs available only by prescription or in dosages that only your doctor can provide. In short, all of the drug options described here must or should be taken only after consultation with your physician.

Since there are many types of arthritis, there are many choices for pharmacologic intervention. Unlike with rheumatoid arthritis or disorders such as psoriatic arthritis, inflammatory bowel disease, and lupus, the pharmacological approach to osteoarthritis is straightforward.

When you meet with your doctor, he or she will discuss with you the treatment alternatives as well as the risks and benefits of each drug. It is essential that you take the prescribed drug as recommended by your physician, since altering the drug regimen cannot only be dangerous but also make the intended treatment less effective. Be sure to report any side effects to your physician immediately.

The major goals of pharmacologic management of osteoarthritis are reduction of pain and inflammation. Drug therapy generally utilizes simple analgesics such as Tylenol or NSAIDs. These over-the-counter medications are used primarily for pain, though the NSAIDs also help control inflammation. I recommend all my patients carefully reserch and read about their medicines on the internet.

Initial Drugs of Choice

In 1995 the American College of Rheumatology published guidelines for treating the more common forms of arthritis of the knee and hip. In general, these guidelines remain relevant today.

The initial drug of choice for arthritis of the hip or knee is acetaminophen, with doses up to 1 gram four times a day. Acetaminophen is a pain reliever and does not decrease inflammation, as it does not have any effects on prostaglandins. Therefore, it does not irritate the stomach or cause gastrointestinal bleeding. However, when taken with alcohol, acetaminophen can cause liver damage.

If a patient does not respond to acetaminophen, then a low dose of an NSAID is recommended, followed by a full dose of an NSAID if appropriate pain relief is not obtained. Like Tylenol, NSAIDs relieve pain, but in addition they reduce inflammation. Because of this dual action, they are, among the most commonly used drugs in our country, with more than seventy million prescriptions written annually. NSAIDs have a relatively low incidence of side effects, yet because they are so widely used, even a relatively uncommon side effect can have a large impact on health care. Therefore, doctors consider all the risks and benefits before prescribing these drugs to patients.

The exact molecular mechanism of pain relief with NSAIDs relates to their ability to inhibit the synthesis of prostaglandins, a group of natural compounds produced in the body that are involved in the generation of pain impulses. NSAIDs also inhibit cellular migrations and interfere with cell processes such as cell binding and membrane permeability, which may contribute to the drugs' anti-inflammatory effects.

There is some question as to whether using NSAIDs to relieve pain and inflammation allows the patient to use the arthritic joint more, thus increasing wear and tear about the articular cartilage. That is, are we possibly doing more harm by masking the pain and reducing the inflammation of joints with NSAIDs? The argument can be made that pain and inflammation are the body's way of signaling the brain, "Hey, I'm hurting here. Do you think we can give up triathlons and do more aqua aerobics instead? If you don't, the little cartilage that we have left is toast."

Scientific theories and musings aside, we know NSAIDs are primarily prescribed for osteoarthritis because of their anti-inflammatory effect. The origin of pain associated with osteoarthritis is not entirely certain and may be related to various causes, including inflammation of the synovium, venous congestion of the underlying bone, stretching of the joint capsule or ligaments with peripheral inflammation, and muscle spasms around the joint. The tissues surrounding the joint are richly impregnated with nerve fibers, while cartilage itself does not have any nerve fibers. Therefore, pain cannot originate from the articular cartilage itself.

The most common side effects of NSAIDs involve gastrointestinal complications. That's why Tylenol—even though it doesn't have the anti-inflammatory advantage of NSAIDs—continues to be wildly popular as a painkiller. The FDA has estimated that approximately two hundred thousand cases of bleeding or perforated ulcers occur each year from NSAID use, and at least a hundred thousand hospitalizations with seven to ten thousand deaths a year can be attributed to their use. That's more than three times the number of people who die from car accidents each year.

Gastrointestinal complications usually surface within the first ninety days of NSAID therapy. Age is positively correlated with bleeding ulcers: patients older than sixty have a risk of complications three times higher than younger patients. A previous gastrointestinal problem also increases risk.

It is unclear whether these risk factors stem directly from NSAID use or if they're associated with other risk factors for peptic ulcer disease, such as smoking, alcoholism, or use of anticoagulant medicines. However, there are medicines that can be taken to help prevent NSAID-induced ulcers. For example, misoprostol, a relatively expensive drug costing $50–$75 a month, has shown to decrease gastrointestinal problems associated with NSAID use.

Kidney problems, which are considered a major toxicity of NSAIDs, are related to the medications' anti-prostaglandin effects. Individuals with preexisting kidney disease and older patients should be monitored for this. Up to 3 percent of patients can develop rashes from taking NSAIDs, and in rare cases NSAID use can lead to liver problems and ringing in the ears. There is also a subtle concern over NSAIDs and cardiovascular risks, including heart attacks and strokes.

Fortunately, NSAID use does not have many other associated drug interactions. However, since many older patients take other medicines, I suggest having a careful consultation with your pharmacist when you are contemplating the use of an NSAID.

Table 7.1 provides a list of over-the-counter and prescription NSAIDs commonly used to reduce pain and inflammation of osteoarthritis. These are powerful drugs with potentially adverse side effects, so even with the OTC NSAIDs, they should be taken only after you have consulted with your doctor.

TABLE 7.1 ANALGESICS COMMONLY USED FOR OSTEOARTHRITIS

BRAND NAME	GENERIC NAME
Advil	Ibuprofen
Aleve	Naproxen
Anacin	Aspirin
Anacin-3	Acetaminophen
Anacin Maximum Strength	Aspirin
Ascriptin	Buffered aspirin
Bayer	Aspirin
Bufferin	Buffered aspirin
Excedrin Extra Strength	Aspirin, acetaminophen
Motrin IB	Ibuprofen
Norwich	Aspirin
Nuprin	Ibuprofen
Panex	Acetaminophen
Tylenol	Acetaminophen
Vanquish	Aspirin, acetaminophen

Analgesics Used Mainly for Pain

- ***Ibuprofen (Addaprin, Motrin):*** Prescription ibuprofen relieves pain, tenderness, swelling, and stiffness caused by osteoarthritis (arthritis caused by a breakdown of the lining of the joints) and rheumatoid arthritis (arthritis caused by swelling of the lining of the joints). It is also used to relieve mild to moderate pain, including menstrual pain.

- ***Naproxen (Aflaxen):*** Prescription naproxen relieves pain, tenderness, swelling, and stiffness caused by osteoarthritis (arthritis caused by a breakdown of the lining of the joints),

(Continues)

**TABLE 7.1   ANALGESICS COMMONLY USED
FOR OSTEOARTHRITIS** (*Continued*)

rheumatoid arthritis (arthritis caused by swelling of the lining of the joints), juvenile rheumatoid arthritis (a form of joint disease in children), and ankylosing spondylitis.

- **Aspirin (prescription):** Prescription aspirin relieves the symptoms of rheumatoid arthritis (arthritis caused by swelling of the lining of the joints), osteoarthritis (arthritis caused by breakdown of the lining of the joints), systemic lupus erythematosus (condition in which the immune system attacks the joints and organs and causes pain and swelling), and certain other rheumatologic conditions (conditions in which the immune system attacks parts of the body).

- **Aspirin (nonprescription):** Over-the-counter aspirin is used to reduce fever and to relieve mild to moderate pain from headaches, menstrual periods, arthritis, colds, toothaches, and muscle aches. Nonprescription aspirin is also used to prevent heart attacks in people who have had a heart attack in the past or who have angina (chest pain that occurs when the heart does not get enough oxygen). Nonprescription aspirin is also used to reduce the risk of death in people who are experiencing or who have recently experienced a heart attack. Nonprescription aspirin is also used to prevent ischemic strokes (strokes that occur when a blood clot blocks the flow of blood to the brain) or mini-strokes (strokes that occur when the flow of blood to the brain is blocked for a short time) in people who have had this type of stroke or mini-stroke in the past. Aspirin will not prevent hemorrhagic strokes (strokes caused by bleeding in the brain). Aspirin is in a group of medications called salicylates. It works by stopping the production of certain natural substances that cause fever, pain, swelling, and blood clots. Aspirin is also available in combination with other medications such as antacids, pain relievers, and cough and cold medications. If you are taking a combination product, read the information on the package or prescription label or ask your doctor or pharmacist for more information.

- **Acetaminophen (Tylenol):** Acetaminophen relieves mild to moderate pain from headaches, muscle aches, menstrual periods, colds and sore throats, toothaches, backaches, and reactions to vaccinations (shots), and to reduce fever. Acetaminophen may also be used to relieve the pain of osteoarthritis.

- **Ketoprofen:** Prescription ketoprofen relieves pain, tenderness, swelling, and stiffness caused by osteoarthritis (arthritis caused by a breakdown of the lining of the joints) and rheumatoid arthritis (arthritis caused by swelling of the lining of the joints). Prescription ketoprofen capsules are also used to relieve pain, including menstrual pain (pain that occurs before or during a menstrual period). Nonprescription ketoprofen relieves minor aches and pain from headaches, menstrual periods, toothaches, the common cold, muscle aches, and backaches, and to reduce fever. It works by stopping the body's production of a substance that causes pain, fever, and inflammation.

Aspirin: Wonder Drug Redux

Aspirin is a truly amazing drug, especially for the treatment of arthritis. It's the original NSAID—a pain reliever with anti-inflammatory benefits. It also can lower fevers and stop you from having a heart attack.

The size of a standard aspirin tablet is 325 mg or 5 grains. Generally, two 5-grain tablets are taken every four hours to obtain pain relief. Some patients have to take twelve to twenty aspirin tablets a day, depending on their body size. Occasionally aspirin can be administered as an over-the-counter extra-strength preparation, which is 500 mg per tablet. Higher doses of aspirin may be needed to decrease inflammation, but this can induce unwanted side effects and therefore should be carefully monitored by your physician. If you experience ringing in the ears (tinnitus), you are taking too much. A simple blood test to measure the salicylate level can ensure that you are taking the correct dosage.

To prevent overdosing, it is imperative that you read the labels on all over-the-counter medications, because many cold medicines, many headache remedies, and some stomach relief medications contain aspirin. When reading labels, look for not just the word *aspirin* but also the terms *acetylsalicylic acid* and *salsalate,* both of which are close relatives of aspirin.

There are medicines that can protect the stomach lining. These include anti-ulcer medicines such as Tagamet (cimetidine) and Zantac (ranitidine) to block stomach acid production. Carafate (sucralfate) coats the stomach lining and can also be used. A new synthetic prostaglandin called Cytotec (misoprostol) is now commonly used to decrease gastrointestinal ulceration and bleeding.

There is no evidence that brand-name aspirin is better than generic brands, but patients can react differently to the different fillers and consistency of different brands, so some brands may be better tolerated than others. Generic aspirin generally costs about a penny per tablet, while the more expensive buffered or enteric-coated aspirins can cost up to 3–5¢ each.

One of the major drawbacks of aspirin is the volume of pills that has to be taken for a beneficial effect. Aspirin is quickly metabolized in the body and stays in the bloodstream for only a short time. Pharmacists use the term *half-life,* which is the time it takes for half of the dose of the drug to be eliminated from the body. Aspirin is known to have a very short half-life, and that is why other NSAIDs with a longer half-life are more commonly used. While many NSAIDs are available only by prescription, ibuprofen (200 mg) and naproxen (220 mg) are available over the counter. These OTC doses are much lower than prescription doses, however, and require many more pills to be taken on a daily basis. Other NSAIDs are generally more expensive than aspirin, though some enteric-coated aspirin approaches the price of other NSAIDs.

NSAIDs are not addictive and do not usually cause sedation or breathing problems. However, it is important to realize that NSAID-related complications often have no prior warning signs, creating potentially serious problems in patients (especially older ones) who take these medicines.

COX-2 Inhibitors: The New Generation of NSAIDs

As I've mentioned, NSAIDs are effective at reducing pain and inflammation because they block the synthesis of prostaglandins. They do this by interfering with a group of enzymes, called cyclooxygenases (COX), that are essential in the production of prostaglandins. Two types of cyclooxygenases, COX-1 and COX-2, are responsible for the production of prostaglandins that cause pain and inflammation. But COX-1 also produces a different type of prostaglandin that protects the stomach and intestinal lining from excessive bleeding. NSAIDs that block both COX-1 and COX-2 interfere with the production of this protective prostaglandin and leave the stomach more vulnerable to gastrointestinal complications.

Recently, however, drug companies have developed a newer category of anti-inflammatory medicines, called COX-2 inhibitors. These newer drugs block only the COX-2 enzyme, not the COX-1 enzymes that are necessary for stomach protection. This allows doctors to treat the pain and inflammation of arthritis without the adverse side effects seen with aspirin and earlier NSAIDs.

There are currently two COX-2 inhibitors on the market. Celebrex (celecoxib) is taken one to two times daily. Mobic (meloxicam) is taken once a day and is approved for use in many countries. (Two other COX-2 inhibitors, Vioxx [rofecoxib] and Bextra [valdecoxib], were taken off the market because of rare but serious side effects.) Some studies suggest that the COX-2 inhibitors may protect us from other diseases such as colon cancer, Alzheimer's disease, and kidney disease.

Narcotics: For Temporary Relief

Arthritis patients with severe pain occasionally need stronger relief, and doctors may prescribe narcotics for this purpose. They are also frequently used after surgery to relieve pain from the operation. Narcotic use will certainly alleviate the pain; however, narcotics can be addictive. This class of drugs should be used only for temporary pain relief. They are certainly not accepted for long-term therapy.

Narcotics work by blocking pain messages to the brain. However, over time the body becomes habituated to the drug, and you need more and more of the narcotic to get the same painkilling benefits. Side effects can include drowsiness, mood changes, and constipation. Excessive use can cause breathing difficulties and even death.

Overall, narcotics should be used sparingly and episodically when there are no other alternatives for short-term pain relief. They should be taken only as directed by your doctor.

A Final Note

Recently an increasing number of drugs designed originally for other purposes are now being marketed for osteoarthritis pain and inflammation. These use a variety of chemicals—some rather unconventional, to say the least.

- **Botox**, that anti-wrinkle sensation, was originally used for migraine headaches and now has still another application: arthritis. Some researchers are experimenting with injections for knee arthritis.

- **Embrel**, a drug for rheumatoid arthritis, is now being marketed for degenerative osteoarthritis.

- **Cymbalta** (duloxetine), an antidepressant, has been tried in an FDA-approved trial for osteoarthritis of the knee.

- **Limbrel**, a flavonoid compound, works on both COX-1 and COX-2 metabolism to help manage osteoarthritis symptoms. It is neither a drug nor a dietary supplement; instead, it is considered a food product that happens to be regulated by the FDA (a first).

- **Osteoporosis drugs such as Protelos** (strontium ranelate) are now being tested for osteoarthritis in England and Germany. Since they strengthen the bone, the thought is they would make the area under the cartilage stronger as well.

Takeaways

There's no drug on the market that restores cartilage; however, a wide range of over-the-counter and prescription drugs are available to relieve the pain and inflammation associated with the cartilage degeneration that occurs in osteoarthritis.

Acetaminophen offers the advantage of effective pain relief while being gentle on the stomach. NSAIDs offer the advantage of reducing both pain and inflammation. COX-2 inhibitors are designed to reduce the potentially harmful side effects associated with earlier NSAIDs. Most NSAIDs (the exception is aspirin) increase the risk of cardiovascular incidents such as strokes and heart attacks. Work with your physician to find the drug that is best for you. Always be familiar with any drug you take and its side effects. Check it out on the internet.

8
ALTERNATIVE ARTHRITIS THERAPIES

A man who smelled like a distillery flopped onto a subway seat next to a priest. The man's tie was stained, his face was plastered with red lipstick, and a half-empty bottle of gin was sticking out of his torn coat pocket. He opened his newspaper and began reading. After a few minutes, the disheveled guy turned to the priest and asked, "Say, Father, what causes arthritis?"

"Mister, it's caused by loose living, being with cheap, wicked women, too much alcohol, and a contempt for your fellow man."

"Well, I'll be," the drunk muttered, and returned to his paper.

A little while later, the priest, having thought about what he had said, nudged the man and apologized. "I'm very sorry. I didn't mean to come on so strong. How long have you had arthritis?"

"I don't have it, Father. I was just reading here that the Pope does."

* * *

The doctor called one of his patients to say, "Mrs. Cohen, your check came back."

Mrs. Cohen answered, "So did my arthritis!"

* * *

A few days after his appointment with an elderly patient, the doctor saw his patient walking down the street with a gorgeous young woman on his arm.

A couple of days later, the doctor spoke to the man and said, "You're really doing great, aren't you?"

The patient replied, "Just doing what you said, Doc: 'Get a hot mama and feel all right.'"

The doctor said, "I didn't say that. I said, 'You've got a heart murmur and arthritis.'"

* * *

Pardon the Henny Youngman humor. But the claims staked out on the Internet for arthritis cures remind me how much of that stuff is a joke. Here's one of my favorite come-hither lines from an Internet promotion: "Cure for osteoarthritis that they don't want you to know about." Put aside for a moment the question of who "they" are or how anyone could keep the cure for osteoarthritis a big secret between them and their million closest friends on the Internet. If you click on this teaser, you're taken to a YouTube video that demonstrates "laser prolotherapy." Essentially, says the video, a "laser light" is passed over your knee, then "light energy is converted to chemical energy" (if Einstein had only known!), and voilà—you're cured. Needless to say, this is a scam. The Arthritis Foundation reports that for every dollar spent annually on legitimate arthritis research, $25 will be spent on unproven remedies.

In this chapter, we'll explore alternatives to standard medical treatments for osteoarthritis. Now, I don't mean to lump all alternative treatments together and say that they're all worthless. Some of the treatments described below are used by legitimate medical professionals, and there may even be studies indicating that a particular treatment may be effective. But other studies may produce conflicting results, and none of the alternatives described here is scientifically proven—at least not yet—to be a long-lasting, effective treatment for osteoarthritis, and certainly not a cure. That said, some of the treatments have received the imprimatur of the insurance industry and in certain circumstances are eligible for coverage.

So approach alternative therapies with a heavy dose of skepticism. Some may work for you, and others won't. Above all, proceed with the greatest caution—some therapies have the potential to do harm. Alternative therapies are like the T-shirt I recently saw on a student at the USC campus: the front said, "It works in practice," and the reverse added, "But does it work in theory?" That is, for some patients alternative therapies may relieve osteoarthritis symptoms, but there's no scientific foundation for their claims.

Placebo Effect

Will an alternative treatment work for you? It may. But it may work in *spite* of the treatment. No doubt you've heard of the placebo effect, where patients given an inert pill or a sham treatment respond as if the ingredients were active. For example, a test subject with arthritis of the hands is told that a new experimental cream contains powerful painkillers, and after trying the cream reports—feels, for all intents and purposes—less pain, even though the cream contains no active ingredients.

Somewhere between 30 and 40 percent of the population seems susceptible to placebo effects, and it is not possible to determine ahead of time whether a placebo will work or not in any given person. Interestingly, the placebo effect works on different physical afflictions to varying degrees. For example, the placebo effect is zero in studies of treatments for blood poisoning, while it shows up to an 80 percent response rate in studies of wounds on the small intestine. With osteoarthritis it's not uncommon to have a placebo effect of 30 percent in scientifically controlled studies

Pain caused by inflamed joints, tendons, and ligaments varies so much in intensity between episodes and between individuals that it's no wonder the placebo effect is relatively high in osteoarthritis treatment. Pain is subjective, and relief is a powerful medicine even if the treatment is a sham.

CLARK STANLEY'S SNAKE OIL
FOR WHAT AILS YOU

The phrase *snake oil* is a derogatory term used to describe quackery, the promotion of fraudulent or unproven medical practices. The term comes from an actual product, Clark Stanley Snake Oil Liniment, which was widely available in the United States in the late nineteenth century.

This is no urban myth—both the man and his product were real. Both came to national prominence during the 1893 World's Columbian Exposition in Chicago, where Stanley captured the public's attention with an exhibit in which he slaughtered hundreds of rattlesnakes, supposedly so that their "snake juice" or oil could be processed. An 1890s advertisement for his patented snake oil liniment promised a "wonderful pain destroying compound" and a "cure of all pain and lameness"—all this plus "immediate relief" for 50¢ (the equivalent of $10 today).

As it turns out, the product itself was lame. When the US Department of Agriculture's Bureau of Chemistry (the forerunner of today's Food and Drug Administration) investigated the product's claims in 1917, it found it was mostly mineral oil with some red peppers to produce heat, and traces of turpentine and camphor to provide its trademark medicinal smell. There was no snake oil or anything of the sort in it, and the whole operation quickly folded.

Stanley was charged with fraud and fined $20. He didn't contest the decision, likely because by that time the self-styled "Rattlesnake King" had made a fortune and was living like royalty. No doubt, too, owing to what we know today about the placebo effect, scores of happy patients would have still bought the product for pain relief for their aching joints if allowed to.

As a footnote, it's not clear where Stanley got the notion of hawking his product as "snake oil," but it probably had something to do with a traditional medicine Chinese laborers who were brought to the United States in the late nineteenth century to build the nation's transcontinental railway used for relief of muscle pain. This remedy was made from a snake native to China. Modern-day analysis confirms that this substance, still used in Chinese herbal medicine today, contains omega-3 fatty acids that in fact can relieve symptoms of stiffness and joint tenderness.

Chiropractic Treatment

Chiropractors believe that through regular joint manipulation the pain of arthritis can be eliminated. They focus on spinal manipulation or spinal adjustments to treat pain. Chiropractors often relieve pain by increasing mobility between spinal vertebrae when the bones have become restricted, scarred, or slightly out of alignment. They can use hand manipulations with gentle pressure, or a specific higher energy as gentle forces, across different joints. You may experience quick relief immediately after manipulation, or it may take weeks to feel the benefit; some treatments may not work at all. Chiropractic treatment may be harmful to individuals with unstable joints, severe osteoporosis, narrowing of the spine (spinal stenosis), or instability of the spine.

It's a good rule of thumb that if you're experiencing severe pain, you should see a medical doctor before going to a chiropractor. Long-term, well-controlled studies have not demonstrated that chiropractic treatment is an effective treatment for osteoarthritis.

Acupuncture

In the last two decades, acupuncture has become popular, and it's even been accepted to a large degree by the medical establishment. (Insurance companies now reimburse for many acupuncture treatments, but not necessarily for osteoarthritis.) Inserting thin-gauge needles in different points of the body causes the release of endorphins, the body's natural stress-relieving hormones. This can lead to a feeling of relaxation and can help decrease the pain of arthritis symptoms. Acupuncture may also trigger release of a hormone that fights inflammation, which is why chronic back pain can be relieved by these treatments. Other studies suggest that a release of hormones such as serotonin creates a calming effect in the body. The National Institutes of Health (NIH) have approved acupuncture for post-op dental pain, nausea during pregnancy, and nausea and vomiting associated with surgery or chemotherapy. The World Health Organization of the United Nations also includes arthritis, lower back pain, sciatica, and tennis elbow as ailments that may benefit from acupuncture.

Treatment may take about twenty minutes, although it can take many treatments to decrease your pain. If you choose to use acupuncture, you should discuss this with your medical doctor. It's best to use a qualified, licensed practitioner of acupuncture.

Biofeedback

Biofeedback is considered an excellent treatment for relaxation and pain relief. It uses electronics to measure body responses associated with stress such as muscle contractions or heart rate. With sensors placed over different areas of your body, you can learn to read tension in your muscles and follow your heart rate and breathing patterns. Monitoring all of these body functions with a trained biofeedback therapist assists you in learning how to relax, which can decrease stress and pain.

Hypnosis

The feeling of calm produced by hypnosis can certainly help individuals cope with the daily pain of osteoarthritis. Proponents believe that focused concentration can help to decrease and control the pain. This is considered a complementary technique to be used in combination with other strategies for pain management, and should be learned from a qualified and certified practitioner.

Prolotherapy

Prolotherapy (not to be confused with "laser prolotherapy," the scam treatment discussed earlier) is the practice of injecting an irritant solution (usually containing dextrose, cod liver oil, phenol, glycerine, or lidocaine) into ligaments and joints to induce an inflammatory response, in order to tighten the joint and stimulate tissue growth. Often available in naturopathy clinics, prolotherapy was first introduced in the United States in the 1930s, but evidence of its effectiveness is inconclusive; consequently, prolotherapy treatment is not covered by most insurance companies.

Still, in theory, those injections should work. We know that in addition to its deleterious effects, inflammation can have a beneficial effect on cartilage. It stimulates substances carried in blood that produce growth factors in the injured area to promote healing. No less than the *New York Times* has written positively about prolotherapy, and the Mayo Clinic has said that if nothing else works, "prolotherapy may be helpful."

Proponents cite experiments—dozens of them since prolotherapy was first studied beginning in the 1950s—in laboratory animals that demonstrated tissue growth in ligaments and tendons stimulated by prolotherapy injections. One study of people with lower back pain showed a 60 percent decrease in the diameter of damaged connective tissue, with patients reporting decreased pain and increased mobility. In another study, patients showed a significant improvement in the symptoms of arthritis in the knee one to three years after prolotherapy injections. A controlled clinical trial sponsored by the National Center for Complementary and Alternative Medicine, part of the National Institutes of Health, is under way. To date, however, there are no evidence-based studies confirming these results.

Interarticular Injections

Interarticular treatment involves entering the knee with needles and injecting one of a number of substances.

Lavage, or washing out a joint, is an option in patients with mild to moderate osteoarthritis. The idea is that injecting sterile fluid into a joint helps wash out much of the interarticular debris and inflammatory chemicals that can cause irritation to the knee. Most studies have shown that, although mildly painful, this treatment does offer some short-term opportunities for relief of osteoarthritis pain; longer-term relief is possible when there are mechanical knee symptoms.

Intra-articular injections of corticosteroids have long been a standard for treatment of arthritis, particularly in the knee. Corticosteroids have a very strong local anti-inflammatory effect, and a new generation of time-release intra-articular steroids recently has come onto the market, allowing the concentration of steroid at the site of the osteoarthritic joint to remain at therapeutic levels for longer periods. However, there is no documentation of long-term benefits with osteoarthritis, and there is some evidence that cartilage can degenerate more quickly with repeated injections. Unfortunately, there have been no standard dosing regimens and no standard preparations of cortisone established to determine what is best for the patients.

Viscosupplementation is the intra-articular injection of hyaluronic acid, a substance that is composed of long chains of carbohydrate molecules and which is present in all the fluids and tissues of the body. Hyaluronic acid is also a major component of synovial fluid and of articular cartilage. In osteoarthritis, the molecules of hyaluronic acid in the synovial fluid shrink, and the concentration of hyaluronic acid in the fluid decreases, which together result in a reduction in the synovial fluid's ability to lubricate the joint and absorb shock. An injection of a hyaluronic-acid-based product into the joint can help restore normal hyaluronic acid concentrations. This treatment was approved by the FDA in 1998. Weekly injections of high-molecular-weight hyaluronic acid have been shown to significantly reduce osteoarthritis pain in the knee.

Currently, there are many commercially available hyaluronic acid therapies: Hyalgan, which consists of five weekly intra-articular injections of a natural form of hyaluronic acid (derived from rooster combs); Synvisc, which is a synthetic form given in three weekly injections (there is now Synvisc-One, a single injection); Supartz, another synthetic form administered as a series of five weekly injections; Euflexa, a synthetic form given as a single injection for three weeks; and Orthovisc, a high molecular weight product made from hyaluronan, given once a week for three weeks. All these preparations have been shown to be as effective as NSAIDs for osteoarthritis in the knee in terms of reducing symptoms, and they can decrease the need for NSAIDs. These improvements persist for several months; side effects are minimal but can include reaction to the injections and ongoing inflammation at the injection sites. The treatments are expensive, however, and there is no evidence that they can reverse the osteoarthritis process.

It has also been suggested that hyaluronic acid injections have positive biochemical effects on cartilage cells, but some placebo-controlled studies have cast doubt on that claim. Generally speaking, hyaluronic acid treatment is recommended primarily as a last alternative before surgery.

Maybe the best evidence that hyaluronic acid injections have "arrived" lies in that benchmark of American entrepreneurialism, the franchise business. Osteoarthritis Centers of America storefront clinics can be found nationwide in communities with lots of wealthy seniors.

PRP

Platelet-Rich Plasma (PRP) is a treatment that uses your own blood as a starting point. A sample of your blood is run through a centrifuge to extract a variety of substances—white blood cells, platelets, growth factor, and others—which are then added to plasma (the liquid part of blood) in various combinations and delivered directly into the joint. There are several different companies and thus different PRP concoctions.

Researchers are excited about PRP because a number of substances in the blood associated with tissue building and repair and with anti-inflammatory effects can decrease inflammation when delivered into the joint. We are not exactly sure how PRP works, but it does appear that it can reduce joint inflammation and thus provide pain relief. We need to quantify the components of these various PRP regimens to get a handle on this new biologic "drug."

This is state-of-the-art stuff, and clinical trials are ongoing. But because this is so new, insurance companies won't cover it, and so patients who want PRP therapy must pay for it out of pocket. Generally, treatments cost $500 to $1,000 each, and so far only a handful of doctors offer it.

Regenokine

Golf legend Fred Couples handily won the prestigious Senior Players Championship in 2012 despite having been sidelined for the past two years with a debilitating arthritic back. Twice named PGA Player of the Year, in 1991 and 1992, Couples joined Jack Nicklaus and Raymond Floyd as the only golfers to win the Players Championship on the regular and senior tours. It's quite the achievement, especially given that Couples essentially had trouble even swinging a golf club just weeks before the tournament because of his condition.

Following the game, Couples revealed in a very public press conference that the secret to his success was a little-known treatment program called Regenokine (the same one that Kobe Bryant had, as I mentioned earlier). "I had the Regenokine treatment, and after just a few weeks I was able to resume my regular playing schedule and I feel fantastic. I have been suffering with back problems for many years, and this treatment has really decreased my pain and allowed me to forget about my back and focus on playing my best. I am feeling better than I have in ten years," he said.

As with other alternative treatments, there are lots of proponents of Regenokine and clinical observations extolling its virtues. There is a randomized clinical trial done in Germany that shows that six injections, over time, decreases pain and improves functions more than the hyaluronic acid and saline injections.

Like PRP, Regenokine uses a small volume of the patient's own blood to derive a concentrated form of an anti-inflammatory protein known as interleukin-1 receptor antagonist (IL-1Ra). This can block the effects of IL-1 on the inflammation process. This makes absolute scientific sense.

The Regenokine treatment falls into a sort of regulatory limbo, which is why it is currently not FDA approved. In a recent article, science journalist Johan Lehrer noted some of the unanswered questions about the safety of Regenokine and other biologic medicines: "Can the blood be heated to a higher temperature, as with Regenokine? Spun in a centrifuge? Can certain proteins be filtered out? Nobody knows the answer to these questions, and most American doctors are unwilling to risk the ire of regulators."

Well, actually, in the United States two clinics—one each in Los Angeles and New York City—skirted around the FDA approval issue by administering Regenokine as an off-label treatment, relying on doctors' established prerogative to essentially prescribe any medicine or treatment deemed helpful to the patient. Only time will tell whether the FDA will allow these doctors to continue this practice (especially in light of the high-profile athletes who have talked about it in press conferences and on TV). In the meantime, Regenokine treatments begin at $5,000 each.

WEARABLE THERAPY

What if the answer to osteoarthritis pain was as simple as slipping on a shirt or pants? A new "therapeutic sportswear line," Evidence Based Apparel (Alignmed), has developed shirts that it claims can immediately correct bad posture, thereby alleviating back pain and increasing mobility. Their pants that do the same for knee pain have been proven to alter the forces at the knee, shifting weight off the painful arthritic portion of the knee.

The formfitting garments use patented "neuro-bands" with precise tensions to stimulate nerves that control muscle movement. When those nerves are triggered, the body fires messages to the brain that induce additional support to the muscles and skeletal structure. The result is a positive anatomic change that can train the body to realign itself, says the manufacturer.

The Evidence Based Apparel line of shirts allows you to move easily in any position without a sense of restriction and can be worn as either outerwear or underwear. (This I can testify to personally.) The manufacturer offers scores of testimonies

(Continues)

WEARABLE THERAPY (*Continued*)

from satisfied customers that the garments reduce or eliminate pain. Former major league baseball pitcher Curt Schilling is among the true believers.

Another, more prosaic form of wearable therapy is Kinesiology Therapeutic Tape (KT Tape). It, too, has been designed to relieve pain and pressure, provide joint support and stability, and increase circulation.

KT Tape is applied along muscles, ligaments, and tendons to provide a lightweight, strong external support. KT Tape works differently for different injuries. It can lift and support the knee-cap, holding it in place, for individuals who have problems with runner's knee. It also can support sagging muscles along the arch of the foot, relieving the connective tissues in individuals who suffer from plantar fasciitis. And it can alleviate biomechanical stress in people who have shin splints, reducing pain and giving the body a better opportunity to recover.

Depending on how it is applied, KT Tape supports, enables, or restricts soft tissue and its movement. By stretching and recoiling like a rubber band, it augments tissue function and distributes loads away from inflamed or damaged muscles and tendons, thereby protecting tissues from further injury.

The tape can stay on for up to three days, but it will loosen with repetitive motions. If you decide to use KT Tape, visit a physical therapist to learn how to properly apply the tape for maximum benefit.

Low Level Laser Light Therapy

Finally, our review of alternative treatments for osteoarthritis would not be complete without a discussion of Low Level Laser Light Therapy. To date, the science behind this technology has been suspect, and it's been used mainly for hair-loss treatments but increasingly for short-term clinical treatment of acute joint pain. While there is anecdotal evidence that it can work in some instances, the science on LLLLT is still out. That, of course, has not stopped the technology from being offered to consumers. The Internet is awash in claims of miraculous therapeutic benefits by "red light" devices that promise, for example, to increase collagen production by "photo-activation."

How does LLLLT work? Well, that's part of the problem. No one knows. It's thought that the laser light somehow stimulates cell metabolism, increases blood flow or disrupts pain transmission by acting on nerves. A recently published scientific study from a Harvard-MIT research group in Boston throws more light, so to speak, on how it might treat osteoarthritis. In a controlled study, the group found inflammation of the cartilage was reduced significantly within 24 hours by a single application of LLLL The researchers hypothesize that its near-infrared photons are absorbed by mitochondria (the part of the cell that creates energy), resulting in an anti-inflammatory effect. Nevertheless, as the authors point out, the study was only with animals, not a clinical study in human disease, and further research is needed to verify the benefits of LLLLT in osteoarthritis.

Takeaways

Like supplements, popular alternative therapies for osteoarthritis run the gamut from the barely plausible to the almost scientific. What's a patient to do? If conventional treatments aren't helping, then explore an alternative therapy. Proceed with caution, especially with therapies such as chiropractic that, if used improperly, carry the risk of damaging tissue and joints. Eastern modalities such as acupuncture have a long history of use, if not scientific proof of their effectiveness.

More recent Western therapeutic innovations involve injecting the arthritic tissue either with painkilling substances or with biologic serums that use a modified form of the patient's own blood to chemically alter the painful inflammation process. High-profile athletes have sworn by some of these biological treatments, but no well-controlled studies exist for proof of their claims.

Alternative therapies appeal to osteoarthritis sufferers who have not found relief through traditional medical approaches to osteoarthritis, such as drugs or surgery, though it is possible at least some of this is a result of the placebo effect.

9
CLINICAL
CASE STUDIES

I divide my professional life among several disciplines: surgery, research, teaching, sports medicine, and clinical practice. I am inspired, informed, and invigorated by each of them. However, my most emotional connections are to the patients who come to see me in my office for their aches and pains. This is stuff that affects the daily lives of ordinary people like you and me, and it's why I became a doctor in the first place.

In this chapter, I'm presenting three case studies of patients taken from my clinical files. The three patients are very different, but they share the common denominator of osteoarthritis. These case studies will demonstrate how the knowledge presented in the preceding chapters can be applied to real-world situations.

The three case studies reflect the three main causes of osteoarthritis: trauma, joint overload, and wear and tear. Interlaced within these are other common factors affecting the severity of the disease, including genetic factors, diet, lifestyle, gender, and other chronic diseases.

If you recognize aspects of yourself in any of the case studies, don't assume that what worked for them will work for you. This is meant as a teaching exercise, not a manual. Certainly, take notes and use them to discuss questions about your own aches and pains with your doctor. However, before you embark on any medical therapy, please consult him or her first.

So I invite you now to come into my office and be a (sterilized) fly on the wall. Our first patient is waiting in reception, and he's getting impatient!

James: Trauma Type

James, twenty-one, is impatient not only to see me but also with life in general. He's a young alpha male who embraces extreme sports with a passion. When he's not snowboarding and skiing in the winter, he's mountain biking in the spring, surfing in the summer, and rock climbing in the fall. He's a natural athlete who doesn't mind falling down in the process of learning his latest sport. He had always quickly bounced back from the scrapes and bruises that came with his extreme recreational lifestyle—until the snowboarding accident.

He had done harder jumps a hundred times before, but this time his board caught an edge and he "hit the knuckle" on his landing. In other words, he jammed his knee.

"Did it hurt?" I asked.

"It sure did, Dr. V. But so what? I've hurt worse before," said James, sitting on the examining table in my office.

This time was different, though. When he got home a few hours after the accident, he was limping. He knew enough about sports injuries to "RICE" his knee—rest, ice, compress, and elevate. It helped for a while, but the hurt came back the next day, and it was worse. I ordered an MRI of his knee, which revealed a tibia plateau fracture with a medial meniscus cartilage tear. It was a serious trauma and needed immediate surgical intervention. We snipped off part of the torn cartilage, put a plate and screws into the tibia to stabilize the fracture, and sewed him back up.

Diagnosis

James's prognosis is good in the short term. He'll be back on the slopes in time for the first snow of the season. But the cold harsh reality is that his long-term prognosis for future knee health isn't so good. Statistically, he now has exponentially increased his risk of developing osteoarthritis in his knee by the time he is middle-aged. Without his meniscus intact, there's less cushioning around his knee joint and increased force on his femur and tibia. What we currently know about the cause of osteoarthritis suggests that the degradation of his fractured articular cartilage probably already has begun, through an undetectable, low-grade inflammation that will gradually build over the next two decades.

On the plus side, there's no history of osteoarthritis in his family, who tend to have above-normal life spans. Genetically, James seems to have won the toss of the coin.

Treatment

After surgery he was on crutches for three months as he worked with a physical therapist to slowly strengthen the muscles around his knee. I had him exercise on a stationary bike for the first few weeks.

In addition to his surgery and physical therapy, what can James do to halt the march toward premature osteoarthritis of the knee? The short answer is to stop participating in sports activities with a high risk of joint injury. It will be tough, but I'm going to do my best to convince him that he can get a thrill from participating in lower-impact sports such as baseball, biking, hiking, swimming, and scuba diving.

Long-Term Prognosis

Later, beginning in his thirties, when many men start to put on weight, James will need to watch his diet to avoid excess pounds that can add additional stress to his damaged knee joint. Luckily, he is a vegetarian now, so if he sticks with it, and with his active lifestyle, he should be able to avoid middle-age spread.

When pain does flare up in his knee, now or in the immediate future, I'll work with him to find the NSAID that's right for him, such as ibuprofen, 600–800 mg when needed (but not more than three to four times a day). I also want him to begin taking 1,500 mg glucosamine and 1,200 mg chondroitin daily. There are no known adverse effects of taking either of these supplements, so my thinking is that we should try to intervene now, given James's high risk of trauma-induced knee osteoarthritis. For the future, if his knee cartilage does prematurely degrade, then I'll explore any emerging anti-arthritis drug therapies or cartilage-preserving treatments as a possible permanent solution.

Erica: Metabolic Type

Erica, forty-nine, has been coming to me for years, ever since she started complaining of bursitis in her elbow when she was in her thirties and still a competitive amateur tennis player. She's a lawyer, and I've seen her career blossom. If you want a helluva good personal injury litigator, you call Erica.

Unfortunately, I've also seen Erica's girth grow with her career. The busier and more successful she became at work, the more sedentary her lifestyle became. Tennis is a distant memory now. Even if she had time, she couldn't handle the game anymore. Standing five feet five inches tall, she now weighs 185 pounds, and her BMI is 30.8, which makes her clinically obese.

As we learned in Chapter 3, Erica is hardly alone with her struggle with weight. Seventy-five million adult Americans—roughly one in three—are clinically obese.

We cleared up the tennis elbow eons ago. However, a few years back, Erica began complaining about stiffness and pain in her hips when she did simple daily activities such as climbing stairs, getting out of her office chair, and even walking for more than a few blocks. She's allergic to NSAIDs, so a daily dose of Tylenol was her painkiller of choice, but even the most powerful over-the-counter dosages were not working that well anymore.

Diagnosis

Her X-rays indicated what I already intuitively knew: she had the beginnings of osteoarthritis of the hip. A pelvic radiograph confirmed the diagnosis. When the hip joint becomes arthritic, the normally smooth cartilage surface is worn away; her cartilage looked more like that of an arthritic woman in her seventies rather than that of someone on the cusp of her fiftieth birthday.

Erica had come to me for prescription-strength Tylenol, but with her diagnosis confirmed, I had something much more comprehensive in mind: nothing less than changing her entire lifestyle. In the process she would change her diet, get back into exercising regularly, and reduce her weight to give her aching hip joints a chance to make it into old age still intact.

For a busy professional, that kind of complete lifestyle change can seem daunting, even impossible. But I was going to ask her to take the necessary steps one at a time. And to help get her on board, I was going to present her lawyerly mind with a hard fact that I thought would impress her: if she didn't change her sedentary ways, she soon would become one of the more than 285,000 Americans annually who undergo a total hip replacement (600,000 Americans undergo a total knee orthoplasty.)

As we'll discuss in detail in Chapter 10, there's no doubt today that osteoarthritis has a genetic component, perhaps accounting for as much as 95 percent of all hip osteoarthritis. Unfortunately, both of Erica's parents have osteoarthritis, and her mother had a hip replacement in her late fifties.

First performed in 1960, hip replacement or total hip arthroplasty is as serious a procedure as they come in orthopedic surgery. Because of the sheer number of hip replacements performed each year, it's tempting to think of the procedure as routine, and statistically it's very safe. But have no doubt: it's serious surgery. It involves removing a diseased hip joint and replacing it with an artificial joint, or prosthesis, consisting of a ball component and a socket made of ceramic, plastic, or metal.

In order to insert a new joint, the damaged bone and cartilage must be removed. First the bone is cut with an electric saw to extract the femoral head. Once the arthritic ball is removed, the worn-out socket can be addressed. Unlike the ball, this bone cannot be cut off because the socket of the hip joint is part of the pelvic bone. Instead, a special tool called a reamer (no kidding) is used to remove the degraded cartilage and bone. You actually can hear the damaged cartilage being removed . . . *scrape, scrape, scrape.*

"Okay, I get it, Your Honor. I promise to change my errant ways. I swear," said Erica, holding up her hand.

"And it can take months to recover," I added. "Did I mention the crutches?"

"Call in the jury. We've reached a final verdict," she laughed. "I will definitely turn over a new leaf if the court could please consider leniency just this once."

Treatment

Traditionally, the goal of therapy for hip osteoarthritis is twofold: relieve pain and preserve the existing function. Now that I had Erica's attention, I was adding a third objective: improve function by decreasing the load on her hips and knees.

To recap, Erica's diagnosis included four of the seven major factors in osteoarthritis:

1. She was in her late forties or older.
2. She was a woman (osteoarthritis is more common in women than in men and more severe, and those trends only increase with age).
3. She was overweight.
4. Her parents had osteoarthritis.

Priority number one was dealing with Erica's weight. Here's what I've learned about helping patients manage their weight: a diet is successful only if it's accompanied by a change in lifestyle. Erica had a superbly analytical mind, so I recommended she read *The Power of Habit* by *New*

York Times reporter Charles Duhigg. The book was chock-full of examples of people who had changed bad habits by following a simple "cue, routine, reward" pattern of behavior. Like Duhigg's own weight problem, which he discusses, Erica's seemed to revolve around her habit of snacking almost unconsciously every afternoon, in her case at the Starbucks conveniently located in the lobby of her high-rise office building. Her usual combo was a double latte with an extra shot of hazelnut syrup and a dessert (the lemon cake was always a good fallback if someone had already snatched the last espresso brownie).

She learned to break her bad routine by substituting a walk around the block for her daily visit to Starbucks. What seemed like a chore at first soon turned into a coveted afternoon break from the pressures of her office. She even stopped to smell the flowers, becoming friends with the florist around the corner and treating herself regularly to a few stems of fresh blooms to grace her desk. She still had her afternoon coffee, but now she made it herself in the office kitchen, using a Starbucks instant coffee packet and low-fat almond milk. I also introduced her to the benefits of eating a whole-food diet low in animal protein, salt, and sugar but high in fresh fruits and vegetables.

These two steps—changing her bad habits and eating a more healthful diet—made all the difference. In nine months she had shed thirty pounds and was well on her way to achieving her ideal weight.

The final step in her lifestyle intervention was getting her body in motion. She joined the local Y, which had a nice big pool, and she began a regular habit (the good kind) of aquatic exercises. (A recent study showed that 70 percent of patients suffering from hip arthritis show marked improvements in pain and function with aquatic therapy.)

Now, you might think Erica would be a good candidate for a regular regimen of glucosamine and chondroitin. While many studies have shown that these two supplements improve the pain and function of arthritic knees, the hips are a different story. The largest trial that focused specifically on hip osteoarthritis, sponsored by the National Institutes of Health, showed those supplements to be no more effective than placebo. In Erica's case, using them probably would have been a waste of money.

Long-Term Prognosis

Someday Erica may need hip replacement surgery. But in the meantime, the lifestyle interventions I've described have effectively slowed the rapid progress of her osteoarthritis. In ten years or so, we'll explore whether Erica is a good candidate for injection of hyaluronic acid into the hip joint. Although this type of injection (also known as viscosupplementation) isn't approved in the United States for treatment of hip osteoarthritis, studies have suggested it reduces pain and improves function, and as her physician, I can prescribe it as an off-label treatment.

Erica is young enough, too, that she might one day enjoy the benefits of genetic therapy for hip osteoarthritis. If indeed she has a genetic predisposition for the disease, a simple blood test would confirm that, and a drug specifically formulated for her personal DNA might not only halt its progress but even reverse its effects by biochemically regenerating her cartilage.

ALL METAL AIN'T HIP

A surge in complaints to the federal government in 2011 has caused most orthopedic surgeons to forswear use of all-metal hip replacements, although they're still available on the market. Once promoted as a breakthrough product, all-metal implants accounted for nearly one-third of the implants in recent years, amounting to hundreds of thousands of devices. But the devices have failed prematurely in thousands of people, shedding tiny particles of metallic debris that can damage a patient's muscle and tissue.

Typically, hip replacement devices last fifteen years; however, the metal-on-metal devices failed en masse after only a few years. Mounting complaints to the FDA—up to five thousand at last count—may signal that the devices will eventually be recalled, possibly becoming the biggest implant problem since a heart device was recalled widely in 2007. The FDA notes that the metal-on-metal hip replacement implants are not life-threatening, but the *New York Times* documented in a recent article that many patients implanted with the devices had suffered crippling injuries.

Most surgeons now implant devices that combine metal and plastic components.

Carl: Wear-and-Tear Type

Carl, sixty-seven, a successful insurance actuary who recently retired, thought that he had absolutely nothing in common with people who like kung pao chicken. He's more of a meat-and-potatoes man himself. But it turns out that the same repetitive motion he used to input figures on a calculator—for what seemed like eight hours a day, five days a week, fifty weeks a year, for almost five decades—is not unlike the repetitive hand motion used to eat with chopsticks.

Over the long haul, any kind of repetitive hand motion can contribute to osteoarthritis. Studies have shown that Chinese and people from other Asian cultures who rely on chopsticks as their primary eating utensils have a higher risk of hand osteoarthritis than people from other cultures. Moreover, the hand used primarily in the pinching maneuvers to eat with chopsticks had the highest incidence of arthritis. To get even more specific, in a study of twenty-five hundred elderly Beijing residents, researchers found that the joint within the thumb that had the most stress pressures was also the most vulnerable to the arthritis.

"No problem, Doc. I won't use chopsticks. I don't even like Chinese food," chuckled Carl, who was sitting in front of my desk, slightly hunched over. "Besides, the pain in my right hand is something I can live with. I take an aspirin every day—it helps with the hand pain, and from what they tell me, it lowers my risk of heart disease, too. What's killing me is the pain in my back."

After a successful career in business and raising three kids, Carl finally was ready for active retirement. He was a workaholic, he admitted, which was why he had delayed his retirement well beyond the time most Americans call it quits. Now he had a bucket list for his golden years, which included travel, gardening, and learning to tango.

Diagnosis

The phrase *morning stiffness* refers to the pain and stiffness patients feel when they first wake up in the morning. That type of all-over pain is common for anyone with osteoarthritis who is sixty or older. And, just as in the vast majority of such cases, Carl's morning arthritis tended to subside about thirty minutes after he started moving around the house and "warming up"—or, more accurately, lubricating his joints through normal body motion.

I wasn't very concerned about the hand osteoarthritis. After all, his days of crunching numbers were behind him now, so he wouldn't have that daily repetitive activity to aggravate the existing cartilage damage in his finger joints. Besides, as he had told me, he already was controlling the pain with an over-the-counter drug.

What I was focused on was his lower back pain. An X-ray confirmed that he had spondylosis, or osteoarthritis of the spine. It is a degenerative disease affecting the spine's facet joints and the intervertebral discs. Osteoarthritis of the spine usually doesn't begin until after the age of forty-five, but it is common after age sixty.

The lower back is the most common location for spinal osteoarthritis, which isn't surprising since the lower back carries most of the weight of the body and is the area of the body that is subject to the most mechanical stress. Excess stress on the lower back can cause back muscle strain as well as irritate spinal joints already damaged by osteoarthritis. It can occur in the neck and upper back as well.

In the early stages of osteoarthritis of the spine there usually isn't any inflammation. By the time pain is felt, irreparable damage to the cartilage between the discs of the spine has already occurred. The space between the vertebrae narrows and bone spurs form. When eventually the bone surfaces rub together, the joints become inflamed. The spine stiffens and becomes less flexible. Carl already was at this stage.

Treatment

Carl had a lot going for him. First, because he was now retired he had the time to really focus on getting better and dealing with his spinal arthritis in a constructive way (rather than just ignoring it the best he could, which had been his MO for the last six or seven years).

"Doc, I kept telling myself if I could just make it to retirement, then things would get better," he said—and I was able to reassure him that they would.

Also on the plus side, he had a keen mind, kept sharp by years of doing financial analysis. He was used to meeting deadlines, and he loved to work.

"That's me. Classic American workaholic," he confessed.

So we were going to use that get-up-and-go gumption to change how Carl thought of osteoarthritis. He was no longer just going to live with it but would tackle it head-on as a project.

But first, a reality check. He had a family history of lower back pain on his father's side of the family. He also had another chronic disease—diabetes (from his mother's side)—that he needed to manage in conjunction with his osteoarthritis. It's not unusual to have more than one chronic disease; more than half of Americans do. He was overweight as well and could stand to lose fifteen to twenty pounds. Keep in mind that every pound of overweight adds between four and ten pounds of force on your weight-bearing joints, depending on the movement. In effect, Carl was experiencing sixty to two hundred pounds of constantly recurring joint pressure that he didn't have to endure.

On the plus side, until recently he had been fairly active in sports, regularly playing softball until a couple of years before, when his back pain had made it impossible.

So, let's recap Carl's osteoarthritis profile:

1. His occupation and posture probably contributed to his disease. The repetitive motion of using his right hand on a calculator and the many long hours spent bent over his desk were likely a cause of his hand and back osteoarthritis. Studies have shown conclusively that bending forward while sitting in a chair results in spinal loading that is several times greater than pressures measured while recumbent or standing. (Increasingly, that's why offices are being designed so that workers can stand at least part of the time to use their computers and answer the phone.) Excessive loading of the spinal discs contributes to increased incidence of disc injury and the cumulative wear and tear that's part of spinal osteoarthritis.

2. He had contributing factors in the form of genetics and multiple chronic diseases. For more than fifty years studies of twins have shown that genetics may be the greatest contributor to spinal osteoarthritis, a factor in perhaps 50 percent or more of cases. And while arthritis and diabetes are not directly related, the diseases often overlap. In fact, recent reports from the Centers for Disease Control found that more than half (52 percent) of people with diabetes also have arthritis. The two diseases have several other commonalities involving chemicals in the body that reduce glucose levels.

3. Age and lifestyle predisposed him to osteoarthritis. By virtue of his sixty-plus years, Carl fell into the age group most likely to experience spinal osteoarthritis. His lifestyle contributed to his lower back pain. He didn't exercise enough (because of the pain) and he was overweight.

With these three markers in mind, we designed a regimen to get Carl moving again so he could enjoy those retirement years that he had earned.

First up, exercise. I suggested he join a tai chi class. Tai chi's slow, gentle rolling movements were a great way to improve Carl's posture and balance without additional pressure on his back. (He also liked the fact that it could be used for mortal combat should the occasion call for it.)

Also, I recommended that Carl try a new product, the "posture shirt" by Evidence Based Apparel. It looks like a stretchy T-shirt, but incorporated into the weave are support bands that touch upon and stimulate key pressure points in the shoulder and back. Professional baseball players swear by it, and now so does Carl. When he's wearing it, his slightly stooped and rounded shoulders are thrust back into perfect posture. He's even playing softball again.

Next on his regimen checklist: weight control. I had no luck in converting him to an exclusively vegetarian diet, but I did convince him to stop eating any salty or sugary snack foods that came in a box and to eliminate all fast foods from his diet. With his new leisure time, he even took a cooking class and began to embrace a Mediter-ranean-style diet, low in animal fat, high in vegetable-based healthy fats such as olive oil, and substituting spices for salt. Over the course of three months, he lost the extra pounds, and his knees thanked him every time he ran to first base.

Finally, it was time to revisit Carl's medication. I switched him to a more powerful NSAID (there are many options) to control the inflam-mation in his back, which enabled him to take a lower dosage of aspi-rin for his heart. I prescribed Celebrex because it has fewer adverse side effects on the digestive tract, and Carl only has to take it once a day.

Long-Term Prognosis

A few years from now, if Carl's spinal osteoarthritis significantly deteri-orates and his pain increases dramatically, we'll explore epidural injec-tions, which are given under local anesthesia. These types of injections, which combine a steroid and an anesthetic, have been proven to relieve intense pain of the lumbar region (the lower part of the spine) when all else has failed.

There's one other, cutting-edge therapy we might explore for Carl: Regenokine, the treatment described in Chapter 8 that uses the patient's own blood to boost natural anti-inflammatory proteins in the joint. I anticipate more of these biologic anti-inflammation drug regimes in the future. If his arthritis back pain continues the worst case scenario is an artificial disk (fairly new process) or a back fusion.

Takeaways

Clinical case studies offer the opportunity to see how applications of various treatments and therapies for osteoarthritis work in the real world. The treatment profile that is best for you will depend on factors such as your age, gender, weight, genetics, and any history of previous joint trauma or other health concerns. Although osteoarthritis is the greatest cause of physical disability in the United States, much of it is self-inflicted. That's good news, because factors such as poor diet and exercise habits can be changed. Waiting in the wings are a host of new ideas about how to treat osteoarthritis, which we'll explore in the final chapters of the book.

10

STEM CELLS: ON THE CUSP
OF THE HOLY GRAIL

Cartilage grows old, gets pitted, deteriorates, and disappears, yet the body needs cartilage for joints to move smoothly. The problem with cartilage is that it's mostly made of water held together with a matrix of scaffolding, and once that scaffolding is damaged, it is difficult to regenerate, because it has very few nerves and a poor blood supply. Why did our body evolve with this flawed design? Nature never anticipated that humans would live so long. Keep in mind that we've nearly doubled the human life span in just a hundred years, largely through advances in conquering bacterial and viral diseases. Like it or not, we're stuck with pre-twentieth-century bodies that, thanks to medical science and technology, are outliving many of their parts.

But what if we could turn back the biological clock and create a whole new batch of fresh cartilage from every patient's own cells? That is the holy grail of osteoarthritis treatment. It's called regenerative medicine and it promises the third great revolution in biotechnology.

The first such revolution, the development of recombinant DNA technology in the early 1970s, allowed for DNA to be cut, spliced, and reassembled in almost any way imaginable. The result was the ability to produce a plethora of lifesaving drugs, including unlimited supplies of safe, synthetic insulin to treat diabetics, human growth hormone to treat a variety of unusual conditions, and the blood-clotting protein known as factor VIII, used to treat hemophiliacs; all of these formerly had to be obtained from natural sources, which made them scarce and carried risks. Recombinant DNA also allowed for the development of the first vaccine for hepatitis B, which affects twelve million Americans and is the most common cause of serious liver infection; unlike other common viruses such as polio, hepatitis B cannot be grown in a lab, so the development of a vaccine had to wait for this new biomedical technology. Finally, recombinant DNA facilitated the development of three widely used methods for diagnosing HIV infection, which helped change AIDS into a chronic condition rather than an inevitably fatal disease.

The second biotech revolution was genomics, a new scientific discipline best known for the mapping of the human genome. Genomics was made possible by advances in computer technology, which allowed for rapid gene sequencing and the manipulation of useful data. I'll talk more in Chapter 11 about how this has facilitated the search for an "osteoarthritis gene."

Regenerative medicine is the third great revolution, made possible by the discovery of embryonic stem cells: human cells that can turn into any other kind of human cell. You may have heard that there's controversy surrounding the use of embryonic stem cells, because of religious and ethical concerns. But science in the last decade has completely sidestepped the issue by devising technology that allows for the use of adult stem cells, which can be made, in effect, to move forward and backward through time.

History of Stem Cell Therapy

The history of stem cell therapy is fascinating, beginning much earlier than almost anyone would guess and featuring missed opportunities, an unlikely worldwide celebrity, shady dealings in the Cayman Islands, and outright fraud.

The theory of stem cells was developed around a century ago by Alexander Maksimov, a Russian-born scientist who gained renown for his work in histology, which focuses on the study of the microscopic anatomy of cells and tissues of plants and animals. His work was cutting-edge stuff in the early twentieth century, just as stem cell therapy is today. Maksimov demonstrated that all blood cells develop from a common precursor cell, confirming the theory of hematopoiesis—in effect, the theory of stem cells in an adult organism.

Despite the blueprint that Maksimov provided, there were no major developments in the field of stem cell research until the early 1960s, when John Gurdon, a young British developmental biologist working at the University of Oxford, successfully cloned a frog using intact nuclei from the somatic cells of a tadpole. At about the same time, two researchers at the Massachusetts Institute of Technology, Joseph Altman and Gopal Das, published a study that indicated there was constant stem cell activity in the brain, but the study was largely disregarded because it went against the long-established belief that adult brains never produced new neurons. Not long afterward, two Canadian researchers, James E. Till and Ernest A. McCulloch, demonstrated the existence of self-renewing cells in the bone marrow of mice. They had produced evidence that Maksimov's theory was correct: stem cells do exist.

Over the next few decades incremental progress was made in discovering stem cells' properties and possible applications. In 1981 Gail R. Martin, at the University of California, San Francisco, showed that embryos could be cultured in vitro and that stem cells could be derived from these embryos; she also coined the term *embryonic stem cell.* In 1988 the first embryonic stem cell lines were created from a hamster; in 1995 the same was done from a primate.

Enter the Clone

And then . . . hello, Dolly! Don't tell me you've already forgotten the first mammal cloned from stem cells. In 1997 Dolly, a Finn Dorset (a Scottish breed of sheep), made the cover of *Time* magazine because she was the first clone produced from a cell taken from an adult mammal, the product of stem cells cultured from the mammary tissue of a sheep. The production of Dolly showed that genes in the nucleus of a mature stem cell are still capable of reverting to an embryonic state—moving back in time, if you will, creating a cell that can then go on to develop into any part of an animal.

Typically Finn Dorsets live until the age of twelve, but only five years after her birth in January 2002, Dolly was diagnosed as having arthritis, a condition usually expected in older animals. She was euthanized a year later because of her severe osteoarthritis and because she had developed a lung disease. A postmortem examination, including a study of her chromosomes, suggested that Dolly might have been susceptible to premature aging: her telomeres (the ends of chromosomes, which are linked to the aging process—telomeres start out long but shorten with age) were shorter than would be expected for a sheep her age. Some even speculated that because she was cloned from the adult stem cells of a sheep six years old, in effect Dolly was already middle-aged when she was born.

A year after Dolly's birth, when she was still so pestered by paparazzi that she had to be kept mostly indoors, an article was published in *Science* magazine documenting how a research team led by University of Wisconsin biologist James A. Thomson had been able to isolate cells from early human embryos and develop the first embryonic stem cells. That discovery opened the door for the practical application of stem cells—universal cells that can turn into any of the body's 230 cell types—and promised to be an important step in humankind's search for treatments for crippling or even fatal diseases.

Throwing a Bioethical Bomb

As the *New York Times* noted later, the discovery essentially threw a "bioethical bomb" into a crowd of vocal religious, scientific, medical, and political figures. The furor arose because Thomson's work involved the destruction of human embryos (the embryos used had been discarded by couples who had had them created for in vitro fertilization but no longer needed them). This aroused the ire of the Catholic Church, evangelical Christian groups, and President George W. Bush, who in 2001 gave a nationally televised speech to announce he was restricting all funding for research on stem cells obtained from human embryos. "At its core, this issue forces us to confront fundamental questions about the beginning of life and the ends of science," he said. "I also believe human life is a sacred gift from our creator." With that, all federal government funding for research on new embryonic stem cells stopped immediately—effectively shutting down stem cell research.

But the debate raged on until 2007, when Thomson reported a new way to turn ordinary human skin cells into what appear to be embryonic stem cells without ever using a human embryo, largely defusing the controversy. (However, scientists still like to have a variety of stem cell lines available—including those from embryos—so they can use the best one for their experiments. Ideally, then, there would be no restrictions whatsoever on the development of stem cell lines.) In a coda to the whole matter, in 2009 President Barack Obama quietly lifted the restriction imposed by his predecessor, making it once again possible for federal funds to be used by scientists working with excess embryonic cells from in vitro fertilization procedures—with one caveat: only research on human embryonic stem cell lines created before 2001 could receive federal funding. To this day, the United States is the only country to impose such a restriction.

In 2004, a South Korean researcher claimed to have produced embryonic stem cells from unfertilized human eggs. If true, the discovery would have made the whole controversy moot. The announcement garnered huge media attention, but unfortunately, the claims were proved to be utterly bogus. However, other fraudulent claims are still being made by clinics worldwide—including some in the United States—that peddle stem cell cures for practically any disease you might have. The FDA rightly cautions consumers to make sure that any stem cell treatment they are considering has been approved by the FDA or is being studied under an FDA-authorized clinical investigation.

In December 2011, three people were arrested in the United States and charged with fifteen counts of criminal activity related to manufacturing, selling, and using stem cells without FDA sanction or approval. According to the indictment, one of the accused, a licensed midwife who operated a maternity care clinic in Texas, obtained umbilical cord blood from birth mothers, telling them it was for "research" purposes. Instead, the midwife sold the cord blood to a laboratory in Arizona, which in turn sent the blood to a paid consultant at a university in South Carolina. The owner of the Arizona laboratory was convicted in August 2011 of unlawfully introducing stem cells into interstate commerce. The consultant, an assistant professor, used university facilities to manufacture stem cell products. He then sent the products back to the Arizona lab, which sold them to a man representing himself as a physician licensed in the United States. The man subsequently traveled to Mexico to perform unapproved stem cell procedures on people suffering from cancer, multiple sclerosis, and other serious diseases. The three defendants allegedly received more than $1.5 million from patients seeking treatment for incurable diseases.

In 2012 the CBS newsmagazine show *60 Minutes* devoted a segment to stem cell fraud, reporting on Internet-advertised stem cell "cures" for multiple sclerosis, ALS (Lou Gehrig's disease), cerebral palsy, Parkinson's disease, and Alzheimer's. Let's be clear: at the present time there are no stem-cell-based cures for these diseases.

The FDA has approved one stem cell product, Hemacord, a cord-blood-derived product manufactured by the New York Blood Center and used in patients with disorders affecting the body's blood-forming system. A second stem cell product, Prochymal, developed by Osiris for graft-versus-host diseases, has not been officially approved by the FDA but has been granted "compassionate use" status on a case-by-case basis. To date, Prochymal has been used primarily for children with graft vs. host disease (GVHD).

Regulation of Stem Cells

The FDA regulates stem cells in the United States to ensure that they are safe and effective for their intended use. Stem cells that come from bone marrow or blood are routinely used in transplant procedures to treat patients with leukemia and other disorders of the blood and immune system.

Umbilical cord blood is collected from a placenta with the birth mother's consent. Cord blood cells are then isolated, processed, and frozen and stored in a cord blood bank for future use. Cord blood is regulated by the FDA, and cord blood banks must follow regulatory requirements. There are many other stem cell products that have been reviewed by the FDA for use in investigational studies. Investigational products undergo a thorough review process as the sponsor prepares to study the safety and effectiveness of the product in adequate and well-controlled human clinical trials. As part of this review, the sponsor must demonstrate to the FDA how the product will be manufactured. The FDA also requires that there be sufficient data generated from animal studies to aid in evaluating any potential risks associated with the use of these products.

What are the risks of using stem cells? If the stem cells have been donated by someone else, they may be contaminated with bacteria or viruses. Even if they're your own, there may be a risk of playing havoc with your own body by inserting cells where biologically they don't belong. Experiments in animals have shown that some stem cells undergo cancerous transformations when transplanted. To date there's no evidence that inserting stem cells into the human body causes cancer, but that's largely because the science is too new. In effect, you are a human guinea pig when you undergo stem cell therapy at this moment in time.

To recap, other than cord blood for certain specified indications, there are no approved stem cell products, and except for the aforementioned treatments for leukemia and other blood disorders or unless you're part of an FDA-approved controlled scientific study (in which case you will be informed fully of the risks), there are no approved stem cell treatments in the United States. So how is it, then, that board-certified doctors in the United States are performing these procedures and claiming they are a cure for osteoarthritis?

NEW STEM PRODUCT FOR
DAMAGED ARTICULAR CARTILAGE

In March 2012 the FDA approved a new treatment called Carticel from Genzyme Biology. The product uses the patient's own articular cartilage cells to treat small areas of damaged knee cartilage that has been caused by repetitive trauma and which previously has not responded to arthroscopic or other surgical repair procedures. I've used it myself on patients, and the results to date are good. But the treatment isn't for arthritis—it's specifically approved for traumatic cartilage lesions, and it isn't approved by the FDA for use in anyone over sixty-five.

Here's how it works. Chondrocytes, or cartilage-generating cells, are removed arthroscopically from a non-load-bearing area of the patient's knee. Those cells are then cultivated in vitro in Boston until they have increased in number by about a hundredfold, at which point they are surgically placed with a second surgical procedure into areas where the patient's articular cartilage has been damaged. These cells are held in place by a small piece of soft tissue from the tibia, called a periosteal flap. The implanted cartilage cells then divide and integrate with surrounding tissue, generating new cartilage. The cost of the treatment ranges from $20,000 to $35,000.

A second-generation technique, called Carticel II, uses a "fleece matrix" implanted with cartilage cells that is arthroscopically inserted into the joint. This procedure is known as matrix autologous chondrocyte implantation and currently is available in Germany, the United Kingdom, and Australia; it will likely be available in the United States soon.

When Doctors Push the Ethical Envelope

Viewers watching the nationally syndicated TV health show *The Doctors* on January 25, 2012, were treated to an upbeat segment about how stem cell therapy purportedly had cured a woman's severely arthritic knee. The segment focused on the Centeno-Schultz Clinic in Colorado, which perhaps more than any other facility utilizes off-label treatments.

The clinic's founders, Drs. Chris Centeno and John Schultz, are more than willing to bask in the limelight. Around the time of the broadcast, the website of their company, Regenexx, proudly stated, "As of March 1, 2012 we have performed more than 3,000 total Regenexx procedures. Approximately 1,300 of these procedures have been bone-marrow derived stem cell procedures (Regenexx-SD and Regenexx-C) on more than 920 distinct patients."

To be clear, both doctors are bona fide MDs. And their procedure of extracting a patient's stem cells from bone marrow, creating a highly concentrated solution that contains million of stem cells by isolating and growing them, and then injecting the cells back into the body is indeed grounded in science. But there is no scientific proof of the stated benefits of these procedures, and the manufacturing process used to create this cell cocktail has not been approved by the FDA.

The shield of off-label use protected the clinic for only a little while. In July 2012, the FDA won a landmark district court case that banned the procedure and reaffirmed the right of the agency to regulate therapies made from a patient's own processed stem cells. The ruling promised to tame the largely unregulated field of adult stem cell treatments in the United States, so without skipping a beat, Centeno and Schultz promptly moved the stem cell part of their operations to the Cayman Islands. Litigation with the FDA continues.

Despite their unorthodox practices, Centeno and Schultz are hardly alone among doctors pushing the professional envelope with their claims for off-label privileges when it comes to stem cell treatments. Just Google "stem cell facelift" and you can see virtually an entire medical specialty—plastic surgeons with credentials from the best medical schools in the country—falling over themselves to offer a procedure with not a shred of evidence to support their claims of benefit. The FDA is vigorously—and sometimes seemingly futilely—attempting to keep abreast of this expanding scientific frontier.

My Unlikely Stem Cell Journey

Orthopedic surgery and stem cell therapy generally don't mix. Orthopedic surgery is all about the physical manipulation and correction of bone, muscle, and connective tissues; when that doesn't work or isn't an option, we cut and remove damaged tissue. I'm unusual in being one of a very few orthopedic surgeons getting involved in the cutting edge of stem cell treatment for osteoarthritis.

It all began with a phone call I received a few years after Randal Mills, CEO of Osiris Therapeutics, a biotechnology company that emerged in the 1990s, had heard me deliver a lecture on tissue banking at a medical conference. Osiris has the distinction of bringing to market the first manufactured drug based on stem cells. Prochymal, currently available in Canada and awaiting FDA approval in the United States, has proven successful in treating children suffering from graft-versus-host disease, a potentially deadly complication of bone marrow transplantation, which is used in leukemia treatment. In some cases the donated stem cells react as if the patient's body is a foreign pathogen and attack vital organs.

Mills was formerly an executive with RTI, a biotech company best known in orthopedic circles for its BioCleanse product—a proprietary solution that safely disinfects cadaver tissue for human transplantation. (I know—shades of Frankenstein's monster and *Night of the Living Dead*. Here's something you may not know: there's an entire network established in the United States for collecting tissue from dead people whose bodies have been donated to science and selling that tissue on the open market. It's all perfectly legal; in fact, it's tightly regulated by the government in order to address safety and ethical concerns. To keep all this cadaver cartilage clean and disease-free, a number of techniques have been used throughout the years. One of the techniques used today, BioCleanse, sterilizes the tissue without breaking down the collagen, a problem with some other methods. Other cleaning and sterilization protocols have been developed as well, all supervised by the American Association of Tissue Banking and enforced by the FDA. See also the sidebar "Facebook and the Cadaver Cartilage Connection" in this chapter.)

When Mills was hired by Osiris, one of the first projects he tackled was the ever-growing need for stem-cell-generated cartilage. There are simply not enough body donations to fill the ever-growing demand of our graying population for high-quality cartilage.

By the time Mills called me I was already primed to move the bar higher in cartilage regeneration. A few years earlier I had visited Sweden to witness autologous chondrocyte implantation, a new surgical treatment for cartilage damage (described in the sidebar "New Stem Product for Torn Cartilage" in this chapter and also in Chapter 6). In this technique, the articular cartilage cells come from the patient's own body, so there is no chance of cell rejection or host-versus-graft disease. The Swedes were well ahead of their American counterparts in experimenting with ACI, having conducted scientifically controlled studies since the 1990s, often in conjunction with American companies, notably Boston-based Genzyme. I became convinced that cartilage transplantation was the future of orthopedics and osteoarthritis treatment in the United States.

Mills offered me the chance to run a double-blind, randomized controlled human trial—the gold standard in scientific studies—for this procedure. My physician colleagues (David Fox, David Dellaero, David Griffin, Jack Farr, and Joel Boyd) and I would explore stem cell regeneration on the most common orthopedic procedures: meniscus tears of the knee.

The study marked the first in which stem cells were actually injected into joints. The fifty-five patients in the study had all had surgery to remove torn meniscus tissue. Osiris processed bone marrow stem cells from donors, which were injected into the patients, who had been divided into three groups. The first group received an injection of 50 million stem cells into the damaged knee cartilage. The second received an even higher dose, 150 million stem cells. The third group was our control group: they received a placebo serum that contained no stem cells. Each group was injected only once and then we followed them for two years, using MRIs given by a team of independent radiologists. Of course, we were all interested in seeing how much meniscus cartilage would be regenerated. However, equally important was determining whether the injections decreased the patient's pain, whether they affected the arthritis present in the knee, and whether they produced any dangerous side effects.

The test subjects in my group were all my patients, some of whom I had been treating for years. They ranged from eighteen to sixty-three years old, comprised both men and women, and came from a wide range of professions. If they had one thing in common, it was that all were athletic to some degree: one was a competitive collegiate swimmer at USC; another was a middle-aged physician and runner from San Francisco. They also shared one other trait: they were selfless in their donation of time to the experiment, and their collective enthusiasm was inspiring.

We completed the two-year study in 2011. The positive results:

- In the two treatment groups actually receiving stem cells, the patients' knee meniscus cartilage increased by as much as 23.5 percent after one year.

- The patients in the stem cell groups also experienced a statistically significant reduction in pain.

- Patients in the placebo group were three and a half times more likely to experience degenerative bone changes associated with osteoarthritis.

- There were no serious side effects from the stem cell injections.

The study also produced one inexplicable result: the statistically significant growth in cartilage recorded after the first year essentially disappeared after two years. In other words, the cartilage gained by the end of the first year was gone—deteriorated—by the end of the second. Why? We will not know until further studies can be done. Perhaps the dosage of stem cells was not high enough. Or perhaps the dosage was fine but the cells needed to be injected over intervals rather than all at once. What we did learn is that the injections relieved pain without compromising the patients' safety, which was absolutely critical in this first-of-its-kind study. I think these stem cells have a strong anti-inflammation effect.

The Future of Stem Cells

What's next in stem cell treatment of osteoarthritis? In the coming five years, expect a steady stream of studies that continue to advance the knowledge that my study and others have already gathered.

The problem with stem cell research is that it is extremely expensive—especially those studies like mine that use humans rather than lab animals—and corporations that might fund such studies are looking at a very long payback period for the investment, if in fact they ever realize any income from it. Like it or not, stem cell therapy is a business comparable to any other, where corporate executives' primary focus is maximizing return on investment for their stockholders. And investors and stockholders don't like to wait.

In 2011, Geron, one of the world's largest biotech companies, pulled the plug on its first-ever human trial of stem cell therapy for spinal cord injuries. The company claimed that it had to make a choice between funding new cancer research and continuing with the stem cell study. Given the number of cancer patients (twenty million) versus spinal cord injury patients (two hundred thousand), the company felt it had to go where the money was.

That decision contrasted sharply with a statement the company's CEO, Thomas B. Okarma, had made two years earlier after approval was granted for the trial. He said then that the study was "the dawn of a new era in medical therapeutics" and placed his company "at the forefront of the medical revolution." The media took the hyperbole one step further by calling it the treatment that could have made Superman walk—a reference to actor and activist Christopher Reeve, best known for his role in the movie *Superman*, who became the face of spinal cord injury victims after an accident left him paralyzed.

The irony is that Geron's study was a success. Its stated goal was simply to establish whether the treatment was safe, and in the four patients injected with Geron's stem cell product, GRNOPC1, there were no ill effects. The disappointment, however, for both patients and Geron management was that the patients had not seen any improvement, even though earlier lab tests using the same basic treatment had given paralyzed lab animals the power to move their hind legs. (You can find on YouTube a video of one of the test animals, a previously paralyzed rat that after receiving essentially the same stem cell treatment was able to walk again.)

To date, no stem cell studies have resulted in companies making any money. In a different time—for example, the Eisenhower-Kennedy-Johnson era of the late 1950s and early 1960s—government funding of such ambitious capital-intensive projects would have been available. But the Great Recession and decreasing political support for such government spending haven't helped. State-initiated funding, such as the California Stem Cell Research and Cures Initiative, a 2004 state ballot measure that funded $3 billion in grants, is a step in the right direction. Still, the noticeable absence of similar initiatives by other states likely means that this was a onetime proposition.

There's also an institutional bias at work. Federal and private grant monies made available for stem cell therapy gravitate toward life-threatening diseases, notably heart disease and cancer. Even though osteoarthritis is a huge drain on the economy—because of its impact on increased health care costs and decreased productivity—and even though osteoarthritis is the most common cause of chronic disability in adults, it still remains in the shadow of stem cell research for other conditions.

One can only wonder what would have happened in the Geron study if more funding had been made available to allow ten or twenty patients, instead of just four, to be injected. (Even for a human trial, four test subjects is awfully paltry.) What if the four patients had been injected multiple times—say, every week? Or what if their dosage had been increased tenfold? The results might have been different.

The study I'm currently working on explores the effectiveness of embryonic stem cells versus adult stem cells (like the kind I used in my previous study). My team and I have had some early indications that cartilage regrowth is greater with embryonic stem cells. This study uses lab animals because a human study is too expensive. My goal is to replicate the study with humans.

Here's what I believe the future holds for stem cell therapy: in the not-too-distant future, maybe ten years, your arthritic knee problems will be resolved or mitigated with an injection, maybe two or more, of stem cells from your own body. Thirty years ago that would have seemed like sheer fantasy, but so would have miniature portable communication and computing devices—now known as smart phones. Already there are lots of clinical observations suggesting that stem cells can improve and in theory regenerate cartilage. The next step is nailing down the science.

Despite all of the current funding problems, the future of stem cell therapy for osteoarthritis is bright. And I look forward to the day when orthopedic procedures will revolve around the test tube rather than the scalpel.

FACEBOOK AND THE
CADAVER CARTILAGE CONNECTION

When you get an orthopedic surgical implant, it comes from a dead body donated to science. All told, about thirty thousand bodies are donated each year for use by surgeons like me. That might seem like a lot of bone grafts cadaver cartilage, but it's not nearly enough.

As you read this, more than 114,000 Americans are waiting for livers, hearts, kidneys, or other organs, and more than 6,000 died waiting in 2011. It's a shocking figure and makes you wonder why more people don't donate their bodies. Nobody knows

(Continues)

FACEBOOK AND THE CADAVER CARTILAGE CONNECTION (*Continued*)

for sure; ethical and religious convictions probably figure into it. Perhaps most people simply don't know about it.

Mark Zuckerberg, the Facebook wunderkind, became aware of the dire need for donated human bodies when his friend Steve Jobs was waiting for a liver transplant. In May 2012 Zuckerberg went on *Good Morning America* to announce a quick and easy way for Facebook users to sign up to become organ donors. By the end of the day, six thousand people had enrolled through twenty-two state registries, according to Donate Life America, which promotes donations and is working with Facebook. On a normal day, fewer than four hundred would sign up.

That's encouraging, but the reality is that we're already doing pretty well when it comes to organ donations per capita. According to the United Network for Organ Sharing, the organization that runs the nation's transplant system, 43 percent of adults in the United States are registered as donors. Unfortunately, donated organs can only be used under certain circumstances, such as when someone has suffered a fatal head injury and temporary use of a ventilator can keep the organs viable. Less than 1 percent of US deaths annually occur under such circumstances.

The limited potential for more organ donors underscores the need for stem-cell-generated human tissue, including cartilage.

Takeaways

The developing science of stem cell therapy offers the holy grail of arthritis treatment—namely, the ability to regenerate new cartilage to replace old cartilage damaged by age, trauma, and disease. One of the wonders of human physiology, cartilage is the perfect organic cushion to protect weight-bearing joints. Yet it has one fatal flaw: unlike some tissue in the human body, notably skin, it cannot regrow itself. Once destroyed, it's gone. Even worse, it's difficult to replace with transplanted new cartilage, and it's hard to keep it in place because of the constant pounding it's subjected to.

In my own stem cell therapy study, patients treated with stem cells experienced a significant reduction in inflamation pain and degenerative bone changes associated with osteoarthritis. The promising future of stem cell therapy for osteoarthritis remains hamstrung by a lack of funding, with precious research dollars more frequently channeled to other chronic diseases. Still, the future for stem cell treatment of OA remains bright as researchers, among them myself, continue to pursue all available avenues.

11

FUTURE THERAPIES:
GENES, BIOLOGICS, TECHNOLOGY

The opening day of USC's football season is always filled with excitement and expectation. The storied Trojans athletic program has produced some of the most celebrated names in Olympic and collegiate sports, and I'm proud to have been associated with the USC athletic department for these extraordinary athletes for the past fifteen years.

Standing on the sidelines, I couldn't also help wondering if these young athletes might be the first to never experience osteoarthritis. If nothing changes in our present circumstances, they and the rest of their generation will have a virtually 100 percent chance of suffering from the disease by the age of seventy-nine. As we discussed in the preceding chapter, the promise of stem cell therapy to treat the disease is just on the horizon now. But what if treatment could be skipped altogether? What if your genetic profile could be read and then altered to remove any risk of osteoarthritis? What if the way to prevent osteoarthritis lies within our own DNA?

It sounds like the stuff of science fiction, but scores of scientists from around the world recently completed a five-year study sponsored by the US National Human Genome Research Institute. The study is called the Encyclopedia of DNA Elements, or ENCODE, and these new discoveries are bringing us tantalizingly closer to finding the gene responsible for osteoarthritis.

Many of my colleagues at USC Keck School of Medicine are involved with genetic studies, and several are in the thick of ENCODE's remarkable research, which revealed that what had formerly been thought of as "junk DNA" is actually a complex network of switches that control how genes function within the cell. When errors or mutations occur in these genetic switches, disease can result. Can we figure out how to manipulate these switches in order to prevent those diseases, including osteoarthritis?

If stem cell therapy is all about regenerating lost cartilage, gene therapy is about preventing the cartilage from being lost in the first place.

Biomarkers

As I've noted, much of the cartilage degradation associated with osteo-arthritis goes undetected until it is too late—once patients feel the pain, the damage is irreversible, at least with conventional therapies. (Some patients never even feel the pain: one seventy-two-year-old patient who had virtually no cartilage left in her right knee came to see me only because of the funny "crunching" sound her knee was making, which was in fact the sound of bone rubbing on bone.) This is one reason osteoarthritis continues to be thought of as a disease of the elderly—by the time most people realize they have it, they're old.

But it's also known that certain destructive cytokines (molecular messengers that regulate the immune system) increase with aging. What if you could take a test when you're, say, thirty-five years old to see if you have a higher-than-average cytokine count or abnomal cytokine interactions? With that knowledge, gene therapy and lifestyle changes could be prescribed to forestall what otherwise would be the inevitability of osteoarthritis in your senior years. Treatment might even consist of a drug designed just for your specific ailment and genetic profile.

While the first great diagnostic tool in the treatment of osteoarthritis was the X-ray, invented in 1893, the new science of biomarkers takes an entirely different approach, using recognition of both normal and abnormal biological processes to indicate where therapeutic drug intervention might be of use. For arthritis, scientists are looking in the blood or urine for products that indicate the breakdown of cartilage.

Currently, there are no reliable or easily measured biomarkers to provide an early diagnosis of osteoarthritis (before a bone, cartilage, or joint defect appears on an X-ray). But there has been a flurry of research in recent years, which parallels the progress made in genomic technologies, such as gene sequencing. In 2011 nearly a hundred scientific papers on biomarkers were published. The Osteoarthritis Research Society International, the leading professional organization focused on osteoarthritis, has even established a "biomarker global initiative" to speed things along.

One type of biomarker test being developed looks at blood tests using a new technique called metabolomics, which analyzes the molecular and chemical processes involved in the body's energy production. One study found that people with osteoarthritis have four or five metabolites that are abnormal in the way certain enzymes function. If the early research can be replicated and extended, a metabolic test may not only indicate your risk of osteoarthritis but also, through reverse engineering of the process that produces the biomarkers, shed light on the mechanisms of the disease itself.

Similarly, proteomics uses emerging technology to catalogue thousands of proteins in blood and joint fluid to identify factors that signal changes associated with the causes of osteoarthritis. In 2012 a Canadian research team announced the identification of two molecules (non-coding RNAs) in blood that were associated with mild cartilage damage in thirty patients who one year previously had undergone orthopedic surgery for an anterior cruciate ligament (knee) injury. Is this the long-awaited biomarker for osteoarthritis? Only time and more studies will tell.

Another study out of Duke University is combining old-school and new techniques to generate some exciting results in predicting osteoarthritis progression. Advanced X-ray imaging, sophisticated protein analysis, and genetic studies are used to identify subsets of patients predisposed to the disease. The team says it can predict with 75 percent accuracy the risk of developing progressive osteoarthritis of the knee over a three-year period. Unlike traditional X-rays, the new advanced imaging monitors changes in texture and composition of joint cartilage and bone.

Gene Therapy

Once we can identify individuals or even subsets of populations who are inclined to osteoarthritis, what then? That's a question that's been on the minds of scientists ever since it was discovered in the 1940s that DNA carries genetic information.

Clearly there is a strong genetic factor in osteoarthritis. In 2004 a large study showed that people with a sibling who already has knee arthritis have double the risk of developing the disease themselves (with men having a slightly greater risk than women). A recent study in Iceland—something of a nationwide laboratory for geneticists because of the historical isolation of its population—confirms this: Icelanders had five times the incidence of hip osteoarthritis as other Scandinavians. Another study indicated that spinal arthritis could have a genetic factor of 65 percent or more. And research has shown that the risk of post-traumatic osteoarthritis after a meniscal tear in the knee is strongly affected by a family history of the disease and, interestingly, by the presence of osteoarthritis of the hand.

So we know that genetics plays a huge role in osteoarthritis. But which gene? That, of course, is the question that the Human Genome Project was supposed to answer. It did . . . and it didn't. As it turns out, there are at least three genes (and maybe as many as nine or more) that seem to be associated with a susceptibility to osteoarthritis.

KEY TERMS IN GENETICS

- **Genes.** Genes are the biological units of heredity. They determine traits such as hair, height, and eye color—and, scientists increasingly suspect, the risk of many, if not most, diseases. Humans have an estimated one hundred thousand genes.

- **DNA.** Genes are composed of very long molecules of deoxyribonucleic acid (DNA), which themselves are composed of individual units called nucleotides (the so-called building blocks of DNA). There are about three billion pairs of nucleotides in the DNA of a typical human cell. Each individual has a "genetic fingerprint" that's a unique, one-of-a-kind nucleotide sequence. (The exception to this rule is identical twins, which are for all intents and purposes clones produced by Mother Nature.)

- **Chromosomes.** Genes are arranged on rodlike structures, called chromosomes, that are composed of DNA and other proteins. In humans, each cell—the basic unit of living organisms—contains forty-six chromosomes (twenty-three pairs), located within the cell's nucleus.

Looking back to when the Human Genome Project was unveiled in 2000, it was probably unrealistic to hope that it would be able to pinpoint a single gene associated with osteoarthritis. Unlike so-called monogenic or homogenous diseases such as cystic fibrosis and sickle-cell anemia, in which there is a mutation in just one gene, osteoarthritis is a term covering a heterogeneous set of diseases. As we learned earlier, a consensus is forming that osteoarthritis is caused in large part by a complex cascade of inflammation factors with various pathways, starting points, and end points, all of which vary among individuals. And people are messy organisms, with bad habits such as eating junk food and smoking, plus overlapping health issues that may include obesity, diabetes, and high blood pressure, making it difficult to tease out genetics' role in this phenomenon.

Despite the challenges of finding the genetic key to osteoarthritis, researchers have homed in on a handful of pathologic pathways that provide intriguing clues. One area of research is focused on certain cytokines, regulatory proteins that are released by cells of the immune system and act as intercellular mediators. One of them, interleukin-1 (IL-1), is particularly involved in osteoarthritis inflammation response and is strongly predictive of osteoarthritis progression. It's thought that if the right delivery system can be found, an appropriate treatment could block inflammation in the synovial fluid and synovial/capsular tissue that surrounds the joint.

Another cytokine that is a major area of research is tumor necrosis factor (TNF), which increases with age. The presence of too much TNF has been implicated in osteoarthritis and rheumatoid arthritis. (On the most basic cellular level, it may turn out after all that the two most prevalent types of arthritis are more related than current thinking allows.) Here, too, we may be able to develop substances to block the effects of this cytokine.

Another line of osteoarthritis gene therapy aims to genetically modify cells to produce positive therapeutic effects. TG-C is an allogenic (donor) cell therapy involving cartilage cells genetically altered to produce a substance called therapeutic growth factor. Cartilage cells stimulated by therapeutic growth factor have demonstrated an important role in the formation of new articular cartilage. A study in Korea is under way with patients who have severe osteoarthritis of the knee, in order to evaluate the safety and effectiveness of this experimental treatment.

Still another treatment may involve a vaccination for osteoarthritis. It may be possible to inject a derivative of IL-1 and TNF that will stimulate the immune system in such a way that "when animals are vaccinated before they develop osteoarthritis, less clinical signs appear when the animals actually develop osteoarthritis. Clinical signs of the disease are suppressed without any severe chronic side effect," as the patent application notes. Possible efficacy in humans has yet to be determined.

Gene therapy in general is a numbers game. Only about a decade ago did we develop the computing power necessary to be able to run the massive quantities of data involved in mapping the human genome. The next phase of gene mapping and sequencing, and the development of resultant therapies, will be aided by next-generation quantum computers that will be far more powerful than anything in use today.

HUMANS VERSUS GUINEA PIGS

The first death of a patient involving an osteoarthritis gene therapy experiment occurred on July 24, 2007. Jolee Mohr, a thirty-year-old Chicagoan who was married and the mother of a five-year-old daughter, fell ill the day after her right knee was injected with trillions of genetically engineered viruses in a voluntary experiment to find out if gene therapy might be a safe way to ease the pain of rheumatoid arthritis. In three weeks she was dead of a massive fungal infection.

The test was designed to produce an anti-inflammatory protein identical to the one in Enbrel, a drug widely used for rheumatoid arthritis and increasingly for osteoarthritis. Mohr, who suffered from rheumatoid arthritis of the knee, took Enbrel and another similar drug called Humira, both of which can leave patients more susceptible to infections.

The FDA eventually ruled that her death was caused not by the experimental drug but most likely by the fungal infection and her suppressed immune system. Yet questions lingered as to why her immune system would suddenly fail after she had been taking both Enbrel and Humira for a long time without incident. An autopsy showed no arthritic damage to her right knee, bringing up the issue of whether she had been misdiagnosed in the first place.

More than eight hundred gene therapy studies involving five thousand US patients have been conducted since the National Institutes of Health approved the nation's first human gene transfer study in 1989. Before agreeing to be a study subject, each participant must be fully informed about and feel comfortable with the risks.

Making Drugs Stick

Developing a genetically engineered drug that is tailored to the patient's specific orthopedic need is only half the problem. Drugs that need to be injected into the joint often must be given frequently because the pharmacologic agent rapidly dissipates. But what if the drug could be induced to stick around longer?

That's the idea behind nanocarrier-mediated drug delivery systems—or nanoparticles. Before a drug is injected into the patient's joint, it is first treated in some way: mixed in with nanoparticles in the form of a gel (synthetic or natural polymers) that encapsulate the active ingredients in the drug, combined with other therapeutic agents such as chondroitin sulfate, or subjected to a combination of the two processes in which an existing therapeutic agent such as hyaluronic acid is cross-linked to carry the new drug in a hydrogel form.

These systems have shown positive results. In one recent study, test results showed that 70 percent of the drug nanoparticles remained in the knee cavity after one week, in contrast to conventional injections in which the drug dispersed within one or two days. Not only do the nanoparticles make drug delivery to the damaged tissue more effective, but they also reduce cost and risk of infection, and they help patients avoid the pain of multiple injections.

The BION-ic Mann

Meeting Alfred E. Mann is an unforgettable experience. This man, who seems at least two decades younger than his eighty-five years, has founded seventeen companies (and counting) without any formal business training, has donated $500 million to various philanthropic ventures, and still works seventy hours a week. He is the embodiment of the self-made man; in another time, Frank Capra would have made a movie about him and cast Jimmy Stewart in the lead role.

My first encounter with him was at his eponymous institute (the Alfred E. Mann Institute for Biomedical Engineering) on the USC campus in Los Angeles. He established his institute in 1998 to bridge the gap between biomedical research and the creation of successful medical products. I was there to see him as a patient (yes, on occasion I make house calls), but also to learn more about a new orthopedic device. During my visit, he fielded calls and staff queries for three or four other projects he has in active development, including an artificial pancreas and a powder insulin inhaler for diabetes (which eliminates the need for injections).

"Dr. Vangsness, my objective is simple. I solve medical problems," he told me. Knowing that he was the first to bring us the rechargeable pacemaker and cochlear implants, I was ready to take notes.

For the next thirty minutes he told me about the BION, an "injectable neuromuscular microstimulator for therapeutic electrical stimulation." Translation: it's a microgadget placed under the skin to stimulate muscle tissue with electrical pulses. In initial studies, 80 percent of the test subjects, who were specifically chosen because they had one of two conditions—post-stroke shoulder disuse atrophy or knee osteoarthritis—showed marked improvement in function and pain, 55 percent for the shoulder and 78 percent for the knee. No swelling was reported where the device was inserted and no uncomfortable sensations were felt. The vast majority of the patients agreed to continue the study after the initial test, and the improvements in their condition continued or got even better.

Muscle weakness is a primary contributing factor to many types of osteoarthritis. When voluntary control of muscles that surround the major joints is impaired because of disease or trauma, connective tissues weaken, increasing pain and immobility. It's why physical therapy and exercise are part of every osteoarthritis health regimen: stronger muscles can help absorb the pounding and vibration that occur every time your foot hits the ground, thus decreasing the force at the knee and minimizing the pain caused by arthritis. But what if you're too weak to exercise? The danger is that the muscle tissue begins to waste away, further restricting mobility and increasing the risk of additional injury.

The device that Mr. Mann held before me was smaller than a paper clip. In fact, the tiny rod could fit within the diameter of a penny and was no thicker than a matchstick. This was the latest iteration of the

BION, and if he had any say in the matter, it soon would be available through a clinic or medical center near you.

It's been well established that electrical stimulation is able to improve muscle strength, especially in situations where peripheral nerves and muscles are intact but underused. Numerous types of neuromuscular electrical stimulators have been developed, but all have had significant shortcomings. Electrodes can be difficult to affix to the skin and can produce an unpleasant prickly sensation because a relatively high electrical current must be passed through the skin. Electrical wires inserted through the skin are painful, cosmetically unappealing, prone to breakage, and a potential conduit for infection. The fully implantable devices available to date are bulky, require clumsy lead wires, and are expensive.

Enter the BION system, which avoids all of the above and includes a software package to allow a physician to recharge the battery and adjust the intensity of the stimulation. At home, patients can use a separate software program to record the time and duration of each session using the device, transferring the information to the doctor's office for discussion when the patient returns for follow-up visits. BIONs are now being produced in small quantities in a lab setting, making it difficult to estimate what their cost might be on the open market. However, their components are relatively inexpensive, so actual cost will likely depend on how many are sold.

3-D Printers and Customizable Body Parts

Biology labs around the world are experimenting with 3-D printers that can actually create living tissue structures. When combined with embryonic stem cells, this technology promises to create a wide range of body parts, from heart valves to knee cartilage. The days of a perennial shortage of fresh, new human tissue to replace old degraded cartilage may be rapidly coming to an end.

Likewise, engineers have created mold-making robotics to customize replacement parts for arthritic damaged tissue right in the operating room. Gone are the days when a patient would have to be satisfied with a one-size-fits-all joint replacement. I've used these remarkable devices myself on patients with early- to middle-stage osteoarthritis, producing on the spot an orthopedic implant that fits like a custom-made glove. Because more of the patient's natural anatomy is preserved and less trauma is inflicted on the knee, patients who undergo this minimally invasive procedure experience better functionality and more natural knee movements, thereby achieving an improved postoperative quality of life.

Biologic Drugs

In the last decade an entirely new type of drug has emerged from research labs: biologic drugs. Biologics are composed of proteins produced by gene-based technology from biological components including living human, animal, or microorganism cells. They contain several thousand atoms and complex structures, unlike the small-molecule structure of chemical drugs.

The drugs Enbrel and Humira were among the first biologics to reach the marketplace; they are typical of this class of drug in that they must be administered by injection rather than by mouth. They're also expensive. But dozens of biologics will be coming off patent in the next few years, which should reduce costs as generic versions come to market. That prospect has the FDA concerned, since biologics are much more complex in structure than conventional medications, making them more difficult to replicate. The FDA already has released regulatory guidelines about three biologics that could pose a health threat to patients and thus require precise screening. Like the original biological substances they mimic, these biosimilars will be injected into specific joints.

A new-generation biologic drug being developed by pharmaceutical giant Merck focuses on a substance called fibroblast growth factor 18 (FGF-18) in the hope of finding a cure for osteoarthritis and acute cartilage damage. This biologic stimulates the formation of new cartilage cells. The growth factor ensures the replenishment of cartilage cells, so that new cartilage matrix can be formed. This gives the body a chance to replace cartilage damaged as a result of osteoarthritis or acute injury with genuine hyaline cartilage, rather than inferior repair cartilage. This in turn can reverse the imbalance between cartilage depletion and cartilage formation that is typical of osteoarthritis.

The therapy involves injecting FGF-18 into the knee, with a treatment cycle consisting of three injections in all, administered at weekly intervals. Two cycles has been the maximum tested so far. To date, Merck has produced three clinical studies: two on osteoarthritis in the knee joint, and one on acute cartilage damage, also in the knee. One of the osteoarthritis studies treated early stages of the disease; the other addressed late ones. These clinical trials were intended to verify the safety of FGF-18 and gain an initial impression of its efficacy. Results should be known in the next few years.

Takeaways

Evidence is overwhelming that there is a genetic influence on osteoarthritis, now estimated to be 65 percent. Gene therapies are aimed at augmenting cartilage and promoting healing by transferring reengineered biologic agents; the ultimate goal is to prevent osteoarthritis in the first place. The most experimental progress has been made with gene transfers to the synovium, the body's natural lubricant that surrounds joints. As it turns out, synovium is a good place for gene therapy to target—it's frequently where the inflammation that leads to osteoarthritis begins, and its tissue is amenable to gene modification.

In particular, research has established a strong association between osteoarthritis and IL-1, one of the key chemicals involved in cartilage and bone destruction. Harnessing and managing IL-1's role as an active player in the inflammation process likely will be the first pathway to a successful genetic treatment for osteoarthritis.

On the other side of the research spectrum, engineers are creating futuristic miniature robotic devices to deliver electrical stimulation to damaged and atrophied muscles, which play a significant role in the pain and loss of mobility associated with osteoarthritis.

Drugs—the original therapy for arthritis, beginning with ancient forms of aspirin—have embraced twenty-first-century technology with a new, genetically engineered class of biosimilars. And bioengineers already have working prototypes of machines that "print" customized living tissue, such as cartilage, muscle, and bone, that one day will be used to patch or even replace arthritic joints.

All of these therapies portend a time in the near future when osteoarthritis will be conquered with treatments personalized to the patient's individual genetic profile or given en masse as a vaccination.

EPILOGUE

Susan is typical of many of my patients: middle-aged, twenty pounds overweight, and beginning to experience prematurely the first symptoms of osteoarthritis, especially in the knees.

When she visited me recently complaining of morning stiffness, I explained to her what was happening—where in her body the inflammation was occurring and why she was experiencing pain. I reviewed some of the options available now for treatment and underscored the importance of lifestyle changes to enhance her arthritis treatment and to improve her overall health.

About five minutes into my monologue, she reached into her handbag, pulled out her smart phone, and sent a text message. When she realized that I had stopped talking, she looked up and sheepishly put the phone away.

"Sorry, Dr. V.! I actually was listening, but that was a lot of information to absorb. You lost me somewhere between NSAIDs and glucosamine. Say, do you have something I could take home and read? Maybe there's a book on this?"

Now it was my turn to be sheepish, because there wasn't one that addressed all the topics on osteoarthritis that I wanted to share with her and all my other patients. So thank you, Susan, for sparking the inspiration for this book.

There's not a doubt in my mind that the epidemic of osteoarthritis will get worse before it gets better. The combination of a graying population and the scourge of obesity, as well as a multitude of other chronic diseases, will cause a dramatic increase in osteoarthritis. My objective with this book is not only to provide individuals with the best information and strategies for dealing with the disease on a personal level but also to make the case for a policy shift that would focus attention on osteoarthritis and channel more funding toward research on the disease.

Earlier I referred to arthritis as a silent epidemic. Despite the fact it is the most common cause of disability and enormously costly to society, only a fraction of available funding goes to osteoarthritis research, compared to research on the other leading chronic diseases. This has to change.

How we offer health care also has to change. In spite of the fact that the United States spends twice as much per capita on health care as any other nation, the level of care we provide is middling. Our life expectancy and infant mortality rates—the two definitive benchmarks of a nation's quality of health care—are well below most of Western Europe's and Japan's. There's no mystery as to why. Because of our market-driven health care system, the United States spends dramatically less on preventive care than other nations. (There's big money in treating chronic diseases with new drugs and equipment, and not so much in preventing them in the first place.) It's estimated that of every dollar spent on medicine in the United States, only 3¢ goes toward prevention.

More money needs to be devoted to educating the public about the dangers of poor diet and lack of exercise. One-third of all Americans are now obese. One-third of all adults do not meet recommendations for aerobic physical activity. If there ever was a correlation that screamed for public education and new public policy initiatives, this is it.

Yes, things will get worse before they get better. But they will get better—that I'm equally confident of. Despite the lack of funding that would expedite new osteoarthritis research, we are on the cusp of a revolution in its treatment. A breathtaking array of new strategies—from stem cells and genetic therapies to bioprinting and nanotechnology—will soon be available for the first time not only to ease the pain and inflammation of osteoarthritis but also to halt and even reverse the effects of the disease.

On the public education front, a new campaign under the auspices of the Osteoarthritis Action Alliance has been launched that is cosponsored by virtually every major organization associated with osteoarthritis: the Arthritis Council, the American Academy of Orthopaedic Surgeons, the Centers for Disease Control, the International Council on Aging, and the National Institute on Disability and Rehabilitation Research, to name a few. This is a focused initiative that aims to achieve three overall goals over the next three to five years:

1. Inform Americans of evidence-based strategies for weight management, including exercise

2. Coordinate an effort to influence public policy on the prevention and management of osteoarthritis

3. Initiate research for successful disease interventions

In its opening salvo, the Osteoarthritis Action Alliance stated that "despite its toll, OA remains a relatively unaddressed public health and economic burden compared to other chronic diseases such as cancer, diabetes and heart." Amen.

Arthritis might be a silent epidemic for now, but that doesn't mean you have to be silent. If you or a loved one suffers from arthritis, fight to be heard by your local and national officials. Pick up the phone, post a letter, send an email, or pay a visit to your mayor, congressional representative, or senator expressing your concern over the lack of attention your government is giving to this disease, which, as we've reported in these pages, most of us are likely to suffer from at some point in our lives.

—*C. Thomas Vangsness, Jr., MD, Los Angeles, 2013*

Acknowledgments

I must acknowledge my mentors from the University of Minnesota, the Hospital for Joint Diseases/NYU, and the Department of Orthopaedic Surgery at the Keck School of Medicine of USC. Medicine is an art form, and I continue to practice this art with the knowledge and collegial support that I have received from these institutions.

I would also like to thank Dan Ambrosio, my editor at Da Capo Press, for his informed and helpful suggestions regarding the title and design of the book, and my literary agent Harvey Klinger for expertly putting the whole project together.

Finally, my thanks go to my editorial collaborator, Greg Ptacek, for his artful wordsmithing, our many breakfast meetings around Los Angeles, his dogged diligence in keeping the project on track, and his laser focus on including only that information ultimately beneficial to the reader.

Glossary

Activities of daily living (ADLs). The activities we normally do in daily living, including feeding ourselves, bathing, dressing, grooming, work, walking, climbing stairs, and sleeping.

Acupuncture. The practice of putting needles into the body for health benefits, such as to reduce pain.

Aerobic exercise. Any exercise that promotes oxygen circulation in the blood (for example, running, cycling, swimming, and in-line skating).

Allergen. A substance, such as pollen, mold, or animal dander, that may produce an allergic reaction.

Alternative medicine. Healing therapies that are usually not scientifically based or proven and generally not taught in medical schools.

ANAs. Antinuclear antibodies. ANAs are found in patients whose immune systems are prone to cause inflammation against their own body tissues. They are associated with a number of autoimmune diseases, such as systemic lupus erythematosus, Sjögren's syndrome, rheumatoid arthritis, polymyositis, and scleroderma.

Ankylosing spondylitis. A rare type of arthritis that causes chronic inflammation of the spine.

Antigen. Something potentially capable of inducing an immune response. Antigens cause formation of antibodies in the body.

Anti-inflammatory. An agent that reduces inflammation without directly antagonizing the agent that caused it.

Apheresis. A technique in which blood is taken, treated or separated, then returned to the donor.

Arteritis, temporal. This rare inflammatory disease of the arteries is also called giant cell arteritis or cranial arteritis and is more common after age fifty. It is detected by a biopsy of an artery and is treated with cortisone. If left untreated, it can lead to blindness or stroke.

Arthritis. Inflammation of a joint that develops into swelling, stiffness, warmth, redness, and pain. There are more than one hundred types of arthritis, the most common being osteoarthritis. Also there are rheumatoid arthritis, ankylosing spondylitis, psoriatic arthritis, lupus, gout, and pseudogout.

Arthritis, rheumatoid. An autoimmune disease characterized by chronic inflammation of the joints that can cause inflammation of tissues in other areas of the body (such as the lungs, heart, and eyes).

Arthrodesis. A surgical procedure that fuses joint bones (the joint) together in a fixed position, commonly performed for pain relief.

Arthroplasty. A surgical procedure that involves reconstruction of a joint using metal, plastic, or ceramic components. It is usually performed for pain relief as well as function.

Arthroscopy. Examination of the inside of any joint through an endoscope, a fiber-optic instrument inserted through a small incision. It is commonly used for diagnosing and treating sports-related injuries or for minor surgical repairs such as removal of small pieces of torn or loose cartilage.

Autoimmune disease. Disease caused by a malfunction of the immune system such that the body appears to attack and degrade its own tissues.

Back pain, low. Pain in the lower back that relates to the bony lumbar spine, discs between the vertebrae, ligaments around the spine and discs, spinal cord and nerves, muscles of the low back, internal organs of the pelvis and abdomen, and skin covering the lumbar area.

Biopsy. Removal of a small piece of living tissue for microscopic examination.

Bone density test. A test for osteoporosis (thinning of the bones), which can lead to fractures and disability.

Bone scan. A test to identify abnormal areas of bone activity, stemming from problems such as fractures, infection, or cancer.

Bouchard's nodes. Bony enlargements in the middle joints in the fingers that may occur in patients with osteoarthritis.

Bursa. A fluid-filled sac that acts as cushion between the muscles, bones, tendons, and ligaments. Its job is to help these tissues slide over each other with less friction. Its lining can release fluid and become inflamed and swollen.

Bursitis. Inflammation of the bursa.

Calcium. A mineral in the body found mainly in the hard part of the bones. Calcium is essential for healthy bones, as well as for muscle contraction, heart action, and normal blood clotting. Food sources of calcium include dairy products, leafy green vegetables such as broccoli and collards, canned salmon, clams, oysters, calcium-fortified foods, and tofu.

Cartilage. Firm, rubbery tissue on the ends of bones in joints, providing a cushion.

Chondroitin. A protein that is a structural component of articular cartilage.

Chronic. Used to describe an illness or problem that lasts a long time, usually three months or more.

Clinical trials. Medical research studies conducted by health care providers. Usually volunteers are recruited into "control groups" and "treatment groups"; those in the latter receive experimental treatments to detect, prevent, or cure medical conditions.

Collagen. The principal structural component of cartilage and other connective tissues. It is a basic protein building block of all tissues in the body.

Complete blood count (CBC). A diagnostic test that measures blood components, including white blood cells, red blood cells, and platelets.

Connective tissue. Tissues found throughout the body that support and connect other tissues and body organs.

Contracture. Stiffness in or around a joint preventing a full range of motion.

Corticosteroid. Any of the steroid hormones made by the cortex (outer layer) of the adrenal gland. Cortisol is a corticosteroid.

COX-1. One of two types of the COX enzyme. It is involved in production of the prostaglandins that help protect the stomach and other organs.

COX-2. The other type of COX enzyme. It is involved in production of the prostaglandins that create inflammation and may be involved in some cancers, such as colon cancer, and in Alzheimer's disease.

CPPD disease. A form of arthritis caused by crystals of a salt called calcium pyrophosphate dihydrate (CPPD) that are deposited in the joints. Pseudogout is one form of CPPD disease.

Degenerative arthritis. *See* **osteoarthritis.**

Degenerative joint disease (DJD). *See* **osteoarthritis.**

Erythrocyte sedimentation rate (ESR). A diagnostic technique that measures inflammation by measuring how fast red blood cells fall to the bottom of a test tube. The red cells fall more quickly if there is currently inflammation going on. Also known as sed rate.

Fibromyalgia (FM). A condition that causes chronic deep muscle pain, stiffness, and tenderness without detectable inflammation in several parts of the body. Fibromyalgia does not cause body damage or deformity. However, undue fatigue plagues 90 percent of patients. Also known as fibrositis or FMS (fibromyalgia syndrome).

Glucosamine. A protein that is a structural component of articular cartilage.

Gout. An arthritic condition characterized by abnormally elevated levels of uric acid in the blood, recurring attacks of joint inflammation (arthritis), deposits of hard lumps of uric acid in and around the joints, decreased kidney function, and kidney stones. The tendency to develop gout and elevated blood uric acid level (hyperuricemia) is often inherited and can be promoted by obesity, weight gain, alcohol intake, high blood pressure, abnormal kidney function, and drugs.

Heberden's node. A knobby enlargement of the joint of the finger, closest to the fingertip, in patients with osteoarthritis. This can be painful.

Human leukocyte antigen (HLA). One of a number of histocompatibility antigens that may be found as genetic markers in patients predisposed to certain forms of arthritis. HLA-B27 is associated with ankylosing spondylitis and Reiter's syndrome. HLA-DR4 is associated with rheumatoid arthritis.

Immune response. Any chemical response by the immune system.

Immune system. The system of organs, tissues, cells, and cell-produced substances that protects the body against pathogens and foreign substances.

Inflammation. Localized redness, warmth, swelling, and pain that result from infection, irritation, or injury.

Inflammatory arthritis. One of the many non-osteoarthritis arthritic conditions, including rheumatoid arthritis, lupus, and others.

Interleukin. Protein chemicals of the body and bloodstream that play a key role in regulating the chemical inflammation process.

Internal medicine. A medical specialty dedicated to the diagnosis and medical treatment of diseases affecting adults. A physician who specializes in internal medicine is called an internist and generally must complete a minimum of seven years of medical school and postgraduate training.

Joint. The structure of the body where two bones come together. The joint allows for motion.

Joint aspiration. Removal of joint fluid with a needle.

Joint capsule. A fibrous capsule that encases the ends of bones and cartilage in a joint.

Juvenile rheumatoid arthritis (JRA). A term used to describe types of inflammatory arthritis that occur in childhood.

Ligament. Thick collagen fibers that connect across and stabilize two bones of a joint. This allows correct alignment between the joints.

Lupus. *See* **systemic lupus erythematosus**.

Lyme disease. A joint infection caused by bacteria transmitted by a tick infesting a large variety of animals, commonly deer but occasionally mice, dogs, and humans.

Magnetic resonance imaging (MRI). A painless non-radiation imaging technique in which large magnets influence the atomic particles of tissue, creating electronic images of the body. Used to distinguish normal from abnormal tissue.

Muscle. Elastic tissues that support the joint and contract in order to allow joint movement.

Myalgia. A self-limiting inflammation of muscles that produces pain, which disappears when the inflammation decreases.

Nodule. A small collection of tissues. The word *nodule* is the diminutive of *node* (meaning "knot or knob"), so *nodule* means "little knot or knob."

Nonsteroidal anti-inflammatory drugs (NSAIDs). Standard medications for the treatment of arthritis that help reduce inflammation and pain but may cause gastrointestinal upset.

Occupational therapist (OT). A licensed practitioner who can evaluate the effect of arthritis on daily activities at home and on the job and help devise ways to perform tasks of everyday living, including prescribing splints and assistive devices for joint movement.

Orthopedics. The branch of surgery broadly concerned with the skeletal system (bones and joints). An orthopedic surgeon is a physician who specializes in surgery of the musculoskeletal system, its joints, and related structures and who must undergo a minimum of five years of additional training after medical school.

Osteoarthritis. By far the most common type of arthritis, caused by inflammation, breakdown, and eventual loss of the cartilage of the joints; also known as degenerative arthritis or degenerative joint disease. It is generally mechanical in origin and caused by trauma or genetics, and thus is different from inflammatory arthritis.

Osteophytes. Small bony formations at the end of joints where cartilage has become degenerated as a result of arthritis.

Osteoporosis. Thinning of the bones, with reduction in bone mass due to depletion of calcium and bone protein; a predisposing factor for fractures.

Osteotomy. A surgical procedure in which the bone is cut and realigned into a better position.

Over-the-counter (OTC). Describes a drug for which a prescription is not needed.

Physiatrist. A physician certified in rehabilitative medicine.

Physical therapist (PT). A licensed professional involved in the physical aspects of medical care, especially the use of exercise and rehabilitation to treat a physical condition. The physical therapist can also prescribe splints, canes, special shoes, and orthotics.

Primary care. The "medical home" for a patient, ideally providing continuity and integration of health care. All family practice physicians, pediatricians, and internists are considered primary care physicians.

Prostaglandin. One of several types of proteins in the body. Some prostaglandins are major contributors to inflammation and pain in arthritis; others serve to protect the stomach and other organs.

Pseudogout. A crystal-induced arthritis similar to gout.

Psoriasis. An inflamed area of skin; may have many causes.

Psoriatic arthritis. A potentially destructive and deforming form of inflammatory arthritis that affects approximately 10 percent of people with psoriasis.

Purine. Basic building blocks of RNA and DNA.

Range of motion (ROM). A quantifiable arc of movement for each joint.

Reiter's syndrome. An inflammation of joints that often follows severe intestinal or genitourinary tract infections. Often called reactive arthritis because the joint inflammation appears to be a reaction to an infection elsewhere in the body.

Rheumatic fever. Systemic illness that usually follows a streptococcal infection; if it is untreated, it may result in a migratory type of arthritis.

Rheumatism. An old-fashioned, imprecise term sometimes used to describe conditions that cause pain and swelling of the joints and the surrounding supporting tissues of ligaments and muscles.

Rheumatoid arthritis (RA). An autoimmune inflammatory disease that causes chronic inflammation of the joints and the tissue around the joints, as well as other organs in the body. The second most common form of arthritis after osteoarthritis.

Rheumatoid factor. An antibody that is measurable in the blood. It is commonly used as a blood test for the diagnosis of rheumatoid arthritis.

Rheumatoid factor is present in about 80 percent of adults (but a much lower proportion of children) with rheumatoid arthritis.

Rheumatoid nodules. Lumps that develop over joint areas that receive pressure, such as knuckles of the hand.

Rheumatologist. An internist who specializes in the diagnosis and treatment of diseases of the bones, muscles, and joints.

Scleroderma. A rash of the rare systemic form of arthritis in which the body produces too much collagen. Excess collagen may be deposited in the skin and other body organs.

Spurs. Bony growths seen in people with osteoarthritis. *See* **osteophytes**.

Steroids. Potent and effective drugs related to the hormone cortisol that quickly reduce swelling and inflammation. *See* **corticosteroid**.

Synovial fluid (joint fluid). A viscous, clear fluid that is produced by the synovial membrane and acts as the lubricant of joints.

Synovial membrane. The lining of the inside of the joint.

Systemic lupus erythematosus (SLE). An inflammatory disease of connective tissue occurring predominantly in women (90 percent of patients). It is considered an autoimmune disease.

Tendon. Strong bands of tissue made of collagen that connect muscle to bone.

Trigger points. Localized areas of tenderness around joints (not joints themselves) that are painful to the touch.

Tumor necrosis factor (TNF). A protein produced in the body that is responsible for influencing inflammation in the joints, including pain, swelling, and the joint destruction common in rheumatoid arthritis.

Uric acid. The product normally present in blood that can result from the breakdown of purines. Excessive accumulation can lead to crystal formation in the joints and gout.

Urinanalysis. A diagnostic test to measure the presence of cells or chemicals in the urine. These can include blood cells and/or proteins.

Bibliography

Altman R, Alarcon G, Appelrouth D, et al. The American College of Rheumatology criteria for the classification and reporting of osteoarthritis of the hip. *Arthritis Rheum.* 1991;34:505–514.

Altman R, Asch E, Bloch D, et al. Development of criteria for the classification and reporting of osteoarthritis. *Arthritis Rheum.* 1986;29:1039–1049.

Altman R, Brandt K, Hochberg M, Moskowitz R, Bellamy N, Bloch DA, Buckwalter J, Dougados J, Ehrlich G, Lequesne M, Lohmander S, Murphy WA Jr, Rosario-Jansen T, Schwartz B, Trippel S. Design and conduct of clinical trials in patients with osteoarthritis: recommendations from a task force of the Osteoarthritis Research Society, Results from a workshop. *Osteoarthritis Cartilage.* 1996 Dec; 4(4):217–243.

Altman RD. Criteria for classification of clinical osteoarthritis. *J Rheumatol Suppl.* 1991;27:10–12.

Altman RD, Gold GE. Atlas of individual radiographic features in osteoarthritis revised. *Osteoarthritis Cartilage.* 2007;15 (suppl A):A1–A56.

Altman RD, Zinsenheim JR, Temple AR, Schweinle JE. Three-month efficacy and safety of acetaminophen extended release for osteoarthritis pain of the hip or knee: a randomized, double-blind, placebo-controlled trial. *Osteoarthritis Cartilage.* 2007;15:454–461.

American College of Rheumatology Subcommittee on Osteoarthritis Guidelines. Recommendations for the medical management of osteoarthritis of the hip and knee: 2000 update. *Arthritis Rheum.* 2000;43:1905–1915.

Aula AS, Jurvelin JS, Toyras J. Simultaneous computed tomography of articular cartilage and subchondral bone. *Osteoarthritis Cartilage.* 2009;17:1583–1588.

Baker KR, Nelson ME, Felson DT, Layne JE, Stano R, Roubenjoff R. The efficacy of home based progressive strength training in older adults with knee osteoarthritis: a randomized controlled trial. *J Rheumatol.* 2001;28:1655–1665.

Bansal PN, Joshi NS, Enterzan V, Grinstaff MW, Snyder BD. Contrast enhanced computed tomography can predict the glycosaminoglycan content and biomechanical properties of articular cartilage. *Osteoarthritis Cartilage.* 2010;18:184–191.

Bekkers JE, Creemers L, Dhert WJ, Saris DB. Diagnostic modalities for diseased articular cartilage—from defect to degeneration: a review. *Cartilage.* 2010;1:157–164.

Bellamy N, Campbell J, Robinson V, Gee T, Bourne R, Wells G. Viscosupplementation for the treatment of osteoarthritis of the knee. *Cochrane Database Syst Rev.* 2005;2:CD005321.

Bellamy N, Campbell J, Robinson V, Gee T, Bourne R, Wells G. Viscosupplementation for the treatment of osteoarthritis of the knee. *Cochrane Database Syst Rev.* 2006 Apr 19;2:CD005321.

Boegard TL, Rudling O, Petersson IF, Jonsson K. Joint space width of the tibiofemoral and of the patellofemoral joint in chronic knee pain with or without radiographic osteoarthritis: a 2-year follow-up. *Osteoarthritis Cartilage.* 2003;11:370–376.

Bondeson J, Wainwright SD, Lauder S, Amos N, Hughes CE. The role of synovial macrophages and macrophage-produced cytokines in driving aggrecanases, matrix metalloproteinases, and other destructive and inflammatory responses in osteoarthritis. *Arthritis Res Ther.* 2006;8:R187.

Brosseau L, Yonge KA, Robinson V, et al. Therotherapy for treatment of osteoarthritis. *Cochrane Database Syst Rev.* 2003;4:CD004522.

Brouwer RW, Jakma TS, Verhagen AP, Verhaar JA, Bierma-Zeinstra SM. Braces and orthoses for treating osteoarthritis of the knee. *Cochrane Database Syst Rev.* 2005;1:CD004020.

Bruyere O, Pavelka K, Rovati CL, et al. Total joint replacement after glucosamine sulphate treatment in knee osteoarthritis: results of a mean 8-year observation of patients from two previous 3-year, randomised, placebo-controlled trials. *Osteoarthritis Cartilage.* 2008;16:254–260.

Burrage PS, Mix KS, Brinckerhoff CE. Matrix metalloproteinases: role in arthritis. *Front Biosci.* 2006;11:529–543.

CDC. Prevalence of disabilities and associated health conditions among adults—United States, 1999. *MMWR.* 2001;50:120–125.

Chevalier X, Jerosch J, Goupille P, van Dijk N, Luyten FP, Scott DL, Bailleul F, Pavelka K. Single, intra-articular treatment with 6 ml Hylan G-F 20 in patients with symptomatic primary osteoarthritis of the knee: a randomised, multicentre, double-blind, placebo controlled trial. *Ann Rheum Dis.* 2010 Jan;69(1):113–119.

Christensen R, Astrup A, Bliddal H. Weight loss: the treatment of choice for knee osteoarthritis? A randomized trial. *Osteoarthritis Cartilage.* 2005;13:20–27.

Clegg DO, Reda DJ, Harris CL, et al. Glucosamine, chondroitin sulfate, and the two in combination for painful knee osteoarthritis. *N Engl J Med.* 2006;354:795–808.

Dahaghin S, Bierma-Zeinstra SM, Ginai AZ, Pols HA, Hazes JM, Koes BW. Prevalence and pattern of radiographic hand osteoarthritis and association with pain and disability (the Rotterdam study). *Ann Rheum Dis.* 2005;64:682–687.

Dieppe PA, Cushnaghan J, Shepstone L. The Bristol OA 500 study: progression of osteoarthritis (OA) over 3 years and the relationship between clinical and radiographic changes at the knee joint. *Osteoarthritis Cartilage.* 1997;5:87–97.

Drovanti A. Therapeutic activity of oral glucosamine sulfate in osteoarthritis: a placebo-controlled double-blind investigation. *Clin Ther.* 1980;3:260–268.

Egger G, Swinburn B. *Planet Obesity: How We're Eating Ourselves and the Planet to Death.* Sydney: Allen and Unwin; 2010.

Ettinger WH Jr, Burns R, Messier SP, et al. A randomized trial comparing aerobic exercise and resistance exercise with a health education program in older adults with knee osteoarthritis: the Fitness Arthritis and Seniors Trial (FAST). *JAMA.* 1997;277:25–31.

Felson DT. Epidemiology of osteoarthritis. In: Brandt KD, Doherty M, Lohmander LS, eds. *Osteoarthritis.* Oxford: Oxford University Press; 2003:9–16.

Felson DT. The verdict favors nonsteroidal inflammatory drugs for treatment of osteoarthritis and a plea for more evidence on other treatments. *Arthritis Rheum.* 2001;44:1477–1480.

Felson DT, Niu J, Clancy M, Sack B, Aliabadi P, Zhang Y. Effect of recreational physical activities on the development of knee osteoarthritis in older adults of different weights: the Framingham Study. *Arthritis Rheum.* 2007 Feb 15;57(1):6–12.

Finucane MM, Stevens GA, Cowan MJ, et al. National, regional, and global trends in body-mass index since 1980: systematic analysis of health examination surveys and epidemiological studies with 960 country-years and 9.1 million participants. *Lancet.* 2011;377:557–567.

Fransen M, McConnell S, Bell M. Therapeutic exercise for people with osteoarthritis of the hip or knee: a systematic review. *J Rheumatol.* 2002;29:1737–1745.

Gabriel SE, Jaakkimainen L, Bombardier C. Risk for serious gastrointestinal complications related to use of nonsteroidal anti-inflammatory drugs: a meta-analysis. *Ann Intern Med.* 1991;115:787–796.

Geenen R, Bijlsma JW. Psychological management of osteoarthritic pain. *Osteoarthritis Cartilage.* 2010;18:873–785.

Gillespie GN, Porteous AJ. Obesity and knee arthroplasty. *Knee.* 2007 Mar;14(2):81–86.

Goldrin MB. The role of the chondrocyte in osteoarthritis. *Arthritis Rheum.* 2000;43:1916–1926.

Grotle M, Hagen KB, Natvig B, Dahl FA, Kvien TK. Obesity and osteoarthritis in knee, hip and/or hand: an epidemiological study in the general population with 10 years follow-up. *BMC Musculoskel Disord.* 2008 Oct 2;9:132.

Guccione AA, Felson DT, Anderson JJ, et al. The effects of specific medical conditions on the functional limitations of elders in the Framingham Study. *Am J Public Health.* 1994;84:351–358.

Hannan MT, Felson DT, Pincus T. Analysis of the discordance between radiographic changes and knee pain in osteoarthritis of the knee. *J Rheumatol.* 2000;27:1513–1517.

Hill CL, Gale DR, Chaisson CE, et al. Periarticular lesions detected on magnetic resonance imaging: prevalence in knees with and without knee symptoms. *Arthritis Rheum.* 2003;48:2836–2844.

Hinman RS, Crossley KM, McConnell J, Bennett KL. Efficacy of knee tape in the management of osteoarthritis of the knee: blinded randomized controlled trial. *BMJ.* 2003;327:135.

Hinman RS, Heywood SE, Day AR. Aquatic physical therapy for hip and knee osteoarthritis: results of a single-blinded randomized controlled trial. *Phys Ther.* 2007;87:32–43.

Hochberg MC, Altman RD, Brandt KD, et al. Guidelines for the medical management of osteoarthritis. I. Osteoarthritis of the hip. *Arthritis Rheum.* 1995;38:1535–1540.

Hochberg MC, Lawrence RC, Everett DF, Cornoni-Huntley J. Epidemiologic associations of pain in osteoarthritis of the knee: data from the National Health and Nutrition Examination Survey and the National Health and Nutrition Examination–1 Epidemiologic Follow-up Survey. *Semin Arthritis Rheum.* 1989;18:4–9.

Hunter DJ, March L, Sambrook PN. Knee osteoarthritis: the influence of environmental factors. *Clin Exp Rheumatol.* 2002 Jan-Feb;20(1):93–100.

Hutley MV, Newham DJ. The influence of arthrogenous muscle inhibition on quadriceps rehabilitation of patients with early, unilateral osteoarthritic knees. *Br J Rheumatol.* 1993;32:127–131.

Interna F, Hazewinkel HA, Gouwens D, et al. In early OA thinning of the subchondral plate is directly related to cartilage damage: results from a canine ACLT-meniscectomy model. *Osteoarthritis Cartilage.* 2010;18:691–698.

International Association for the Study of Obesity, International Obesity Task Force. Global obesity prevalence in adults. www.iaso.org /site_media/uploads/Prevalence_of_Adult_Obesity.

Jordan KM, Arden NK, Doherty M, Bannwarth B, Bijlsma JW, Dieppe P, Gunther K, Hauselmann H, Herrero-Beaumont G, Kaklamanis P, Lohmander S, Leeb B, Lequesne M, Mazieres B, Martin-Mola E, Pavelka K, Pendleton A, Punzi L, Serni U, Swoboda B, Verbruggen G, Zimmerman-Gorska I, Dougados M. EULAR Recommendations 2003: an evidence based approach to the management of knee osteoarthritis: report of a task force of the Standing Committee for International Clinical Studies Including Therapeutic Trials (ESCISIT). *Ann Rheum Dis.* 2003 Dec; 62(12):1145–1155.

Kahan A, Uebelhart D, De Vathaire F, Delmas PD, Reginster JY. Long-term effects of chondroitins 4 and 6 sulfate on knee osteoarthritis: the study on osteoarthritis progression prevention, a two-year, randomized, double-blind, placebo-controlled trial. *Arthritis Rheum.* 2009 Feb;60(2):524–533.

Kellgran JH, Lawrence JS. Radiological assessment of osteo-arthrosis. *Ann Rheum Dis.* 1957;16:494–502.

Kerrigan DC, Lelas JL, Goggins J, Merriman GJ, Kaplan RJ, Felson DT. Effectiveness of a lateral-wedge insole on knee varus torque in patients with knee osteoarthritis. *Arch Phys Med Rehabil.* 2002;83:889–893.

Kirkley A, Webster-Bogaert S, Litchfield R, et al. The effect of bracing on varus gonarthrosis. *J Bone Joint Surg Am.* 1999;81:539–548.

Lachance L, Sowers M, Jamadar D, Jannausch M, Hochberg M, Crutchfield M. The experience of pain and emergent osteoarthritis of the knee. *Osteoarthritis Cartilage.* 2001;9:527–532.

Lane NE, Gore ER, Cummings SR, et al. Serum vitamin D levels and incident changes of radiographic hip osteoarthritis: a longitudinal study. *Arthritis Rheum.* 1999;42:854–860.

Lane NE, Lin P, Christiansen L, et al. Association of mild acetabular dysplasia with an increased risk of incident hip osteoarthritis in elderly white women: the Study of Osteoporotic Fractures. *Arthritis Rheum.* 2000;43:400–404.

Lanyon P, O'Reilly S, Jones A, Doherty M. Radiographic assessment of symptomatic knee osteoarthritis in the community: definitions and normal joint space. *Ann Rheum Dis.* 1998;57:595–601.

Laupattarakasem W, Laopaiboon M, Laupattarakasem P, Sumananont C. Arthroscopic debridement for knee osteoarthritis. *Cochrane Database Syst Rev.* 2008 Jan 23;(1):CD005118.

Lementowski PW, Zelicof SB. Obesity and osteoarthritis. *Am J Orthop* (Belle Mead, NJ). 2008 Mar;37(3):148–151.

Lievense AM, Bierma-Zeinstra SA, Verhagen AP, Bernsen RM, Verhaar JAS, Koes BW. Influence of sporting activities on the development of osteoarthritis of the hip: a systematic review. *Arthritis Rheum.* 2003;49:228–236.

Lievense AM, Bierma-Zeinstra SM, Verhagen PA, van Baar ME, Verhaar JS, Koes BS. Influence of obesity on the development of osteoarthritis of the hip: a systematic review. *Rheumatology* (Oxford). 2002;41:1155–1162.

Lin J, Zhang W, Jones A, Doherty M. Efficacy of topical non-steroidal anti-inflammatory drugs in the treatment of osteoarthritis: meta-analysis of randomised controlled trials. *BMJ.* 2004;329:324–326.

Lo GH, LaValley M, McAlindon T, Felson DT. Intra-articular hyaluronic acid in treatment of knee osteoarthritis: a meta-analysis. *JAMA.* 2003;290:3115–3121.

Lobstein T, Baur L, Uauy R, for the IASO International Obesity Task Force. Obesity in children and young people: a crisis in public health. *Obes Rev.* 2004;5 (suppl 1):4–104.

Loeser RF. Aging and osteoarthritis: the role of chondrocyte senescence and aging changes in the cartilage matrix. *Osteoarthritis Cartilage.* 2009 Aug;17(8):971–979.

Loughlin J. The genetic epidemiology of human primary osteoarthritis: current status. *Expert Rev Mol Med.* 2005;7:1–12.

Maillefert JF, Hudry C, Baron G, et al. Laterally elevated wedged insoles in the treatment of medical knee osteoarthritis: a prospective randomized controlled study. *Osteoarthritis Cartilage.* 2001;9:738–745.

Manheimer E, Cheng K, Linde K, et al. Acupuncture for peripheral joint osteoarthritis. *Cochrane Database Syst Rev.* 2010;1:CD001977.

Marijnissen AC, Vincken LK, Vos PA, et al. Knee Images Digital Analysis (KIDA): a novel method to quantify individual radiographic features of knee osteoarthritis in detail. *Osteoarthritis Cartilage.* 2008;16:234–243.

May S. Self-management of chronic low back and osteoarthritis. *Nat Rev Rheumatol.* 2010;6:199–209.

Mazzuca SA, Brandt KD, Buckwalter KA, Lequesne M. Pitfalls in the acuate measurement of joint space narrowing in semiflexed anteroposterior radiographic imaging of the knee. *Arthritis Rheum.* 2004;50:2508–2515.

McAlindon T, Formica M, LaValley M, Lehmer M, Kabbara K. Effectiveness of glucosamine for symptoms of knee osteoarthritis: results from an Internet-based randomized double-blind controlled trial. *Am J Med.* 2004;117:643–649.

McAlindon TE, Gulin J, Felson DT. Glucosamine and chondroitin for treatment of osteoarthritis of the knee or hip: a systematic quality assessment and meta-analysis. *JAMA.* 2000;283:1469–1475.

McAlindon TE, Snow S, Cooper C, Dieppe PA. Radiographic patterns of osteoarthritis of the knee joint in the community: the importance of the patellofemoral joint. *Ann Rheum Dis.* 1998;57:595–601.

McCarthy CH, Callaghan MJ, Oldham JA. Pulsed electromagnetic energy treatment offers no clinical benefit in reducing the pain of knee osteoarthritis: a systematic review. *BMC Musculoskel Disord.* 2006;7:51.

McConnell S, Kolopack P, Davis AM. Western Ontario and McMaster Universities Osteoarthritis Index (WOMAC): review of its utility and measurement properties. *Arthritis Rheum.* 2001;45:453–461.

Messier SP, Legault C, Mihalko S, Miller GD, Loeser RF, DeVita P, Lyles M, Eckstein F, Hunter DJ, Williamson JD, Nicklas BJ. The Intensive Diet and Exercise for Arthritis (IDEA) trial: design and rationale. *BMC Musculoskel Disord.* 2009 Jul 28;10:93.

Moseley JB, O'Malley K, Petersen NJ, et al. A controlled trial of arthroscopic surgery for osteoarthritis of the knee. *N Engl J Med.* 2002;347:81–88.

Moskowitz RW. Nutraceuticals as therapeutic agents in osteoarthritis: the role of glucosamine, chondroitin sulfate, and collagen hydrolysate. *Osteoarthritis.* 1999;25:379–395.

Murphy L, Schwartz TA, Helmick CG, Renner JB, Tudor G, Koch G, Dragomir A, Kalsbeek WD, Luta G, Jordan JM. Lifetime risk of symptomatic knee osteoarthritis. *Arthritis Rheum.* 2008 Sep 15;59(9):1207–1213.

Nevitt MC, Xu L, Zhang Y, et al. Very low prevalence of hip osteoarthritis among Chinese elderly in Beijing, China, compared with whites in the United States: the Beijing Osteoarthritis Study. *Arthritis Rheum.* 2002;46:1773–1779.

Nuñez M, Nuñez E, del Val JL, Ortega R, Segur JM, Hernandez MV, Lozano L, Sastre S, Macule F. Health-related quality of life in patients with osteoarthritis after total knee replacement: factors influencing outcomes at 36 months of follow-up. *Osteoarthritis Cartilage.* 2007 Sep;15(9):1001–1007.

Oakley SP, Portek I, Szomor A, et al. Arthroscopy—a potential "gold standard" for the diagnosis of the chondropathy of early osteoarthritis. *Osteoarthritis Cartilage.* 2005;13:368–378.

Oka H, Muraki S, Akune T, et al. Fully automatic quantification of knee osteoarthritis severity on plain radiographs. *Osteoarthritis Cartilage.* 2008;16:1300–1306.

Oliveria SA, Felson DT, Reed JI, Cirillo PA, Walker AM. Incidence of symptomatic hand, hip and knee osteoarthritis among patients in a health maintenance organization. *Arthritis Rheum.* 1995;38:1134–1141.

O'Reilly SC, Jones A, Muir KR, Doherty M. Quadriceps weakness in knee osteoarthritis: the effect on pain and disability. *Ann Rheum Dis.* 1998;57:5888–5894.

Paradowski PT, Englund M, Lohmander LS, Roos EM. The effect of patient characteristics on variability in pain and function over two years in early knee osteoarthritis. *Health Qual Life Outcomes.* 2005 Sep 27;3:59.

Pelletier JP, Martel-Pelletier J, Abramson SB. Osteoarthritis, an inflammatory disease: potential implication for the selection of new therapeutic targets. *Arthritis Rheum.* 2001;44:1237–1247.

Powell A, Teichtahl AJ, Wluka AE, Cicuttini FM. Obesity: a preventable risk factor for large joint osteoarthritis which may act through bio-mechanical factors. *Br J Sports Med.* 2005 Jan;39(1):4–5.

Recnik G, Kralj-Iglic V, Iglic A, Antolic V, Kramberger S, Rigler I, Pompe B, Vengust R. The role of obesity, biomechanical constitution of the pelvis and contact joint stress in progression of hip osteoarthritis. *Osteoarthritis Cartilage.* 2009 Jul;17(7):879–882.

Reginster JY, Deroisy R, Rovati LC, et al. Long-term effects of glucos-amine sulphate on osteoarthritis progression: a randomised, pla-cebo-controlled clinical trial. *Lancet.* 2001;357:251–256.

Richette PJ, Pointou C, Garnero P. Beneficial effects of massive weight loss on symptoms, joint biomarkers, and systematic inflammation in obese patients with knee OA. *Ann Rheum Dis.* 2011;70:139–144.

Roddy E, Zhang W, Doherty M. Aerobic walking or strengthening exer-cise for osteoarthritis of the knee? A systematic review. *Ann Rheum Dis.* 2005;64:544–548.

Sellam J, Berenbaum F. Clinical features of osteoarthritis. In: Firestein GS, Budd RD, Harris ED Jr, McInnes IB, Ruddy S, Sergent JS, eds. *Kelley's Textbook of Rheumatology.* Philadelphia: Elsevier Inc.; 2008;1547–1561.

Sellam J, Berenbaum F. The role of synovitis in osteoarthritis. *Nat Rev Rheumatol.* 2010;6:625–635.

Shakibaei M, Csaki C, Mobasheri A. Diverse roles of integrin receptors in articular cartilage. *Adv Anat Embryol Cell Biol.* 2008;197:1–60.

Sharma L, Dunlop DD, Cahue S, Song J, Hayes KW. Quadriceps strength and osteoarthritis progression in malaligned and lax knees. *Ann Intern Med.* 2003;138:613–619.

Sharma L, Sung J, Felson DT, Cahue S, Shamiyeh E, Dunlop DD. The role of knee alignment in disease progression and functional decline in knee osteoarthritis. *JAMA.* 2001;286:188–195. [Erratum: *JAMA.* 2001;286:792].

Sharp JT, Angwin J, Boers J, et al. Computer based methods for mea-surement of joint space width: update of an ongoing OMERACT project. *J Rheumatol.* 2007;34:874–883.

Teichtahl AJ, Wluka AE, Proietto J, Cicuttini FM. Obesity and the female sex, risk factors for knee osteoarthritis that may be attributable to systemic or local leptin biosynthesis and its cellular effects. *Med Hypotheses.* 2005;65(2):312–315.

Torres L, Dunlop D, Peterfy C, et al. The relationship between specific tissue lesions and pain severity in persons with knee osteoarthritis. *Osteoarthritis Cartilage.* 2006;14:1033–1040.

Towheed TE, Maxwell L, Judd MG, Catton M, Hochberg MC, Wells G. Acetaminophen for osteoarthritis. *Cochrane Database Syst Rev.* 2006;1:CD004257.

Van Klooster R, Hendriks EA, Watt I, Kloppenburg M, Reiber JH, Stoel BC. Automatic quantification of osteoarthritis in hand radiographs: validation of a new method to measure joint space width. *Osteoarthritis Cartilage.* 2008;16:18–25.

White House Task Force on Childhood Obesity. Solving the problem of childhood obesity within a generation. Washington DC, 2010. www.lets move.gov/sites/letsmove.gov/files/TaskForce_on_Childhood _Obesity_May2010_FullReport.pdf (accessed June 23, 2011).

Wise BL, Niu J, Zhang Y, et al. Psychological factors and their relations to osteoarthritis pain. *Osteoarthritis Cartilage.* 2010;18:883–887.

Witt CM, Jena S, Brinkhaus B, Liecker B, Wegscheider K, Willich SN. Acupuncture in patients with osteoarthritis of the knee or hip: a randomized, controlled trial with an additional nonrandomized arm. *Arthritis Rheum.* 2006;54:3485–93.

Yusuf E, Nelissen RG, Ioan-Facsinay A, Stojanovic-Susulic V, DeGroot J, van Osch G, Middeldorp S, Huizinga TW, Kloppenburg M. Association between weight or body mass and hand osteoarthritis: a systematic review. *Ann Rheum Dis.* 2010 Apr;69(4):761–765.

Zhang W, Doherty M, Arden N, et al. EULAR evidence based recommendations for the management of hip osteoarthritis: report of a task force of the EULAR Standing Committee for International Clinical Studies Including Therapeutics (ESCISIT). *Ann Rheum Dis.* 2005;64:669–681.

Index